SOCIAL PHARMACY
Innovation and Development

SOCIAL PHARMACY
Innovation and Development

Edited by

Geoffrey Harding
Department of Public Health Sciences,
St. George's Hospital Medical School, University of London

Sarah Nettleton
Department of Social Policy and Social Work,
University of York

Kevin Taylor
Department of Pharmaceutics
School of Pharmacy, University of London

London
THE PHARMACEUTICAL PRESS
1994

Copies of this book may be obtained through any bookseller or, in any case of
difficulty, direct from the publisher or publisher's agents:
    The Pharmaceutical Press
    (Publications division of the Royal Pharmaceutical Society of Great
    Britain)
    1 Lambeth High Street, London SE1 7JN, England

Australia
    The Australian Pharmaceutical Publishing Co. Ltd.
    40 Burwood Road, Hawthorn, Victoria 3122, and
    Pharmaceutical Society of Australia
    Pharmacy House, P.O. Box 21, Curtin, ACT 2605

Germany, Austria, Switzerland
    Deutscher Apotheker Verlag
    Birkenwaldstrasse 44, D-7000 Stuttgart 1

Japan
    Maruzen Co. Ltd.
    3–10 Nihonbashi 2-chome, Chuo-ku, Tokyo 103

New Zealand
    The Pharmaceutical Society of New Zealand
    124 Dixon Street, P.O. Box 11640, Wellington 1

U.S.A.
    Rittenhouse Book Distributors, Inc.
    511 Feheley Drive, King of Prussia, PA 19406

ISBN: 0 85369 322 6

Typeset by Books Unlimited (Nottm), Rainworth NG21 0JE. Printed and
bound by The Cromwell Press Ltd, Broughton Gifford, Melksham, Wiltshire

CONTENTS

CONTRIBUTORS

Pierre Aïach is a Sociologist and Directeur de Recherche, Institut National de la Sante et de la Recherche Medicale, Villejuif Cedex, France

Nick Barber is Professor of the Practice of Pharmacy, School of Pharmacy, University of London

Marina Barnard is Senior Research Fellow, Centre for Drug Misuse Research, Glasgow University

Ian Bates is Lecturer in Pharmacy, School of Pharmacy, University of London

Ros Batty is Principal Pharmacist, North Thames (West) Regional Clinical Pharmacy Unit, Northwick Park Hospital, Middlesex

Elizabeth Beech is Principal Pharmacist, North Thames (West) Regional Clinical Pharmacy Unit, Northwick Park Hospital, Middlesex

Kerstin Bingefors is Associate Professor, Division of Social Pharmacy, Uppsala University, Sweden

Alison Blenkinsopp is Director of the Centre for Pharmacy Postgraduate Education, Manchester

Wendy Bottero has recently completed her Ph.D. in the Department of Sociology, University of Edinburgh

Nicky Britten is Lecturer in Medical Sociology, United Medical and Dental Schools of Guy's and St. Thomas's Hospitals

Dominique Cèbe is a Sociologist and Ingenieur de'Etude, Institut National de la Sante et de la Recherche Medicale, Villejuif Cedex, France

Sarah Cunningham-Burley is Lecturer in Medical Sociology, Department of Public Health Sciences, Medical School, University of Edinburgh

Peter Davis is Senior Lecturer in Medical Sociology, School of Medicine, University of Auckland, New Zealand

Justin Greenwood is Reader in Public Administration, The Robert Gordon University, Aberdeen

Geoffrey Harding is Senior Research Fellow, Department of Public Health Sciences, St. George's Hospital Medical School, London

Owen Hargie is Professor of Communication, University of Ulster at Jordanstown

Ivor Harrison is Lecturer in Clinical Pharmacy, Welsh School of Pharmacy, Cardiff

Dag Isacson is Associate Professor, Division of Social Pharmacy, Uppsala University, Sweden

Neil McKeganey is Director, Centre for Drug Misuse Research, Glasgow University

Norman Morrow is Director of Postgraduate Pharmaceutical Education and Training for Northern Ireland

Sarah Nettleton is Lecturer in Social Policy, Department of Social Policy and Social Work, University of York

Rhona Panton is Professor of Pharmacy Policy and Practice, Keele University

Kay Roberts is affiliated to the Medicines Research Unit, Welsh School of Pharmacy, Cardiff

Elizabeth Robinson is Senior Lecturer in Psychology Practice, University of Birmingham

Janie Sheridan is a Boots Teacher/Practitioner based in the Department of Pharmaceutics, School of Pharmacy, University of London

Felicity Smith is Lecturer in Pharmacy Practice, School of Pharmacy, University of London

Kevin Taylor is Lecturer in Pharmaceutics, School of Pharmacy, University of London

David Webb is Teacher/Practitioner based in the Department of Pharmaceutics, School of Pharmacy, University of London

FOREWORD

Just as we learned earlier this century that it would not be sufficient to educate pharmacists to prepare elegant dosage forms, we are recognising once again that society requires a pharmacist in the near future with different skills and abilities. It is an outstanding opportunity presented to us with the publication of *Social Pharmacy: Innovation and Development* by Harding, Nettleton and Taylor. The editors have provided us with a resource for self-instruction and with a vehicle within faculties of pharmacy for serious study in the realm of Social Pharmacy.

And it is the discipline of Social Pharmacy that can be the driving force behind the future prowess of our profession. In essence, robots can count tablets more accurately and at less expense than humans, technicians can compound medications in pharmacies and huge, automated factories can do likewise. Persons without professional education at University are able to sell drugs and to serve as cashiers. Yet in the near future, there will be a need for a person who understands the overall health care delivery system, who can serve as a health educator, gatekeeper, referral agent, problem solver and coordinator. Such an individual must be comfortable with interpersonal communication, understand a bit of psychology and sociology and be a problem solver. The pharmacist of the future will offer the missing hand-holding function now disappearing, as society is forced to deal with interactive computer technology in banking, contacting airlines and other services by telephone, as well as the lack of human contact as catalogue and mail catalogue shopping increase in popularity. Similarly, the growth of self service shopping further exacerbates this vacuum.

Into this void steps the new pharmacist, educated of course in pharmacology. pharmaceutics, phathophysiology and pharmacotherapeutics, but one who also understands and knows how to employ the placebo effect, how to perform an intervention in the name of medication adherence (compliance), and a person who is able to work on incentives, understanding the principles underlying the health belief model, and who is an empathetic, caring professional.

If we look very carefully, not into the future, but rather only at today, we find that the drugs that will become available early in the 21st century are in the drug company laboratories today, and with few exceptions there are no awesome advances over contemporary therapies. This is an analogous situation when considering surgery. However one area where some progress can be expected within the decade is in that of behavioural medicine. The sooner the better we learn that diet, and drinking, smoking, lack of exercise and stress can play significant and potentially very negative roles in our health status. No one is more easily accessible than the community pharmacist. He or she may be consulted long hours every day, without an appointment, and without expense. When pharmacy educators and association leaders recognize this, then serious planning for our future roles may begin. This book is one such tool along that road to professional justification and preparedness for a future, strong, viable profession.

The chapter by Nettleton and her co-editors explaining the concept of Social Pharmacy is a valuable one even for readers with only a passing interest in this domain. Bates and his colleagues have hit the nail on the head when they offer teaching strategies for today. Several of the the following chapters provide insight into the work and challenges in pharmacy and the chapter on French Pharmacy is an excellent source of reinforcement or a reminder that our problems are neither unique nor insoluble.

The description of Social Pharmacy in Sweden offers the reader interesting contrasts and lessons. The other chapters dealing with care for special groups or subcultures are fascinating and provide us with both interesting information and a wealth of researchable questions. For this individual, I found myself absolutely captivated by the Pharmacy Primary Care chapter by Smith, and by the work on communication by Hargie and Morrow. Both help explain the vast and valuable opportunity for tomorrow's pharmacist in the provision of primary care services.

By taking Social Pharmacy seriously within the profession and by making an effort to understand its role, we can gain insight and perspective that should be able to guide us in the direction of fulfilling patient needs and expectations in the future. We have had a difficult choice until now for even if we understood the critical and vital importance of Social Pharmacy, there were precious few places to turn to obtain materials, to prepare ourselves.

However, now that we have this book available, there can be few excuses why one has not directed one's own personal attention to this area in an organized fashion. This is not a sermon, but we must take advantage of this situation.

It may be most convenient and comfortable for us to continue to emphasize pharmacognosy or material medica, but there will be plenty of time to do this if the profession does not embrace the skills and competencies in Social Pharmacy and learn how to use these teaching in actual patient care situations.

Thanks to Harding, Nettleton and Taylor, we now have a means to prepare for present and future pharmacist provided services.

Albert I. Wertheimer, B.S. Pharm., M.B.A., Ph.D.

Vice President, Pharmacy/Managed Care

FIRST HEALTH Services Corporation

Previously:

Dean, Philadelphia College of Pharmacy and Science

Richmond, Virginia

December, 1993

ACKNOWLEDGEMENTS

The editors wish to thank Graham Florence of the Computer Unit, School of Pharmacy, and Jennifer Taylor, of the Department of Public Health Sciences, St George's Hospital Medical School, University of London for computing support. Our thanks are also due to Felicia Emmanuel of the Jocelyn Chamberlain Unit, St George's Medical School, for secretarial assistance.

Chapter 11 was originally published in the *British Journal of Addiction*. A slightly revised version is published here by permission of Carfax Publishing Co.

CHAPTER ONE

THE CONCEPT AND CONTEXT OF SOCIAL PHARMACY

Sarah Nettleton, Geoffrey Harding and Kevin Taylor

Health care workers not only treat disease but strive to prevent it. To do this effectively, they cannot rely exclusively on biomedical explanations of health and illness, because the antecedents of health and illness reside not solely within the body, but also beyond it; in the social and physical environment. Commensurately, public health strategies towards illness prevention and health promotion are increasingly targeting individual lifestyles and recognising the need for social and environmental change. Therefore, health care services and practitioners are now concerned not only with disease and treatment, but also with health and the promotion of wellbeing. Thus, as the context in which pharmacy is practised changes, so too does its image and nature, and pharmacists are increasingly recognised as key players in health care delivery. Their role extends beyond the dispensing of drugs, to incorporate provision of advice to clients, negotiating with other health workers about medications and therapies, and contributing to the provision of a more cost-effective health service. Pharmacists' work is now increasingly varied and socially complex. Yet how pharmacists operate within their social and political environment – the basis of social pharmacy – remains a relatively unexplored area of health work.

SOCIAL PHARMACY

Although well established elsewhere, particularly in the USA and Scandinavian countries, social pharmacy is a relatively recent concept within Britain, often subsumed under the generic term "Pharmacy Practice"[1]. Initially it was synonymous with the demography of medicines use and "pharmacoepidemiology" but its remit now extends well beyond drug-use surveillance. Social pharmacy has developed as a hybrid: drawing on methodologies and theories from the social and behavioural sciences in order to explore a diverse range of topics within pharmacy practice. What constitutes social pharmacy will therefore depend on the objects or topics of interest, so that its boundaries will be constantly changing and evolving. In this respect, it is perhaps best thought of as a field of study which draws upon on a range of disciplines to examine and understand matters which are pertinent to the practice of pharmacy.

Nevertheless, social pharmacy is potentially distinct from those disciplines (such as sociology, politics, psychology and economics) which contribute to it. After all, the prime goal of social pharmacy is to understand and illuminate matters of concern to pharmacy. We can therefore distinguish between the topic of social pharmacy and the discipline of social pharmacy. In this respect social pharmacy is akin to other fields of study such as social policy[2] or health promotion[3]. Whilst they clearly form identifiable and distinct disciplines, they are also eclectic in origin and are dependent on other related disciplines for the pursuit of their goals.

Given the interdisciplinary nature of social pharmacy it is necessary for its practitioners to be familiar with the range of relevant disciplines and to appreciate their methodologies. Indeed, a recognition of this need formed one of the main motivations for this edited collection. It aims to provide, through the use of illustrative studies, both an overview of, and an insight into, a number of disciplines which are of value to the study of social pharmacy. Reflecting this aim, contributions are drawn from researchers in several disciplines: sociology, psychology, political science, educational studies, communications and pharmacy practice. This not an exhaustive list of disciplines relevant to social pharmacy, and the potential contribution of other disciplines, such as economics, history and anthropology, should not be underestimated.

The issues addressed in this text are diverse, but they all illuminate matters of pivotal importance to contemporary practice of pharmacy. The variety of the research topics and questions addressed in the book is mirrored by the broad range of methodologies employed. This is inevitable given that the methods of investigation should, to a significant extent, be determined by the research questions the study seeks to address. It is hoped therefore, that those with an interest in the practice of pharmacy will find the text informative, not merely in terms of the findings of the research which are presented (which will of course contribute to social pharmacy's growing and distinctive body of knowledge), but also as a resource.

Qualitative and quantitative research methods, both represented in this volume, are fundamental to the study of health care and its social context. The selection of a given method will invariably depend on the aims and purposes of the research and must be appropriate and suitable to it.[4] If it is perceptions, meanings and experiences which the researcher seeks to illuminate then qualitative approaches are essential, as is clear from the contributions by McKeganey and Barnard and Cunningham-Burley (Chapters 11 and 6).

However, if the aim is to demonstrate changing prescribing patterns on a national scale (see Davis, Chapter 12), or to describe the changing gender composition of the profession of pharmacy (see Bottero, Chapter 3) then quantitative analyses are more suitable. Very often good research combines both approaches to provide a fuller understanding of the problem at hand.

THE CHANGING CONTEXT OF PHARMACY

Social pharmacy has appeared at a time of significant social change which has facilitated the emergence of, and created a need for, this discipline. In Western industrialised nations there have been major demographic, economic and political changes which have impacted on the nature and delivery of health care. For example, change has occurred in the form of aging populations which command different forms of health and social care. The disease burden has also shifted from acute to chronic conditions, which again has implications for the type of health care that is appropriate. Economic changes have had dramatic effects on health care expenditures, which in turn remain inflationary and seemingly uncontainable. Political changes have witnessed a growth in consumer movements and recipients of health care who seek to have a say in the type of treatment that they receive. In relation to health and medicine there has also been a significant shift, in that the biomedical model no longer holds sway. The limitations of the biomedical model, which for so long dominated Western medicine, have been well documented[5] and now the need for a socio-environmental approach to health care is widely accepted[6]. Of course the contribution of social and environmental factors have been recognised within the field of public medicine since the nineteenth century, but at that time public health was concerned with matters such as sanitation, water, and hygiene. Many of the proponents of environmental reforms were not medical practitioners, and public health has, until relatively recently, remained marginal to medicine itself. Indeed, the discipline of social medicine was only established during the 1940s in Britain, and the status of social medicine, community medicine and public health medicine has been, to say the least, shaky in relation to its parent discipline.[7]

Today however, the picture is somewhat different. The "New Public Health", with its emphasis on the impact of social and behavioural factors on health and wellbeing is being hailed, by policy makers and health professionals alike, as the way forward to improve the health status of the nation.[8] The promotion of health, rather than simply the treatment of disease, is now being recognised as a crucial aspect of both health policy and of the daily activities of all health workers.

The curricula of a range of health professions have over the years developed in accordance with these trends. The sociological and psychological aspects of health have been taught in medical schools since the 1970s. Nurses' training now incorporates the study of the social and behavioural sciences and dental schools are also increasingly teaching the sociological, as well as the psychological, aspects of dental health. Pharmacy education is no exception, although formal endorsement of social and behaviourial science teaching within the pharmacy curricula was only given by the Nuffield Committee in their 1986 report on the future of pharmacy.[9] Thus socio-economic, cultural and political factors are now, more than ever, recognised within health professions' curricula as equally important constituent determinants of health states as those of bio-pathology. The impact of these factors on health states are addressed in the pharmacy undergraduate curricula and form the basis of "social pharmacy".

INNOVATION AND DEVELOPMENT

Innovations and development in social pharmacy, form the cornerstone of this book. The chapters are diverse in their focus and subject matter, however they describe development and innovations that have occurred because of the changing socio-cultural and political context in which we live. Recurrent themes in this volume include: interdisciplinarity; professionalisation; education and communication and efficiency and effectiveness in health service delivery. Moreover, many of these themes are transnational, as contributions from authors extending from the United Kingdom to France, Sweden, USA and New Zealand illustrate.

Interdisciplinarity

Social pharmacy is not unique in applying methods from a range of disciplines to specific problems. Turner, in a discussion of interdisciplinarity in medicine, has noted that:

> 'Interdisciplinarity has emerged in a context where it is claimed that contemporary health (or more general social) problems cannot be tackled on a monodisciplinary basis; the interdisciplinarity debate is tied therefore to the quest for effective problem solving.'[10]

As we have already indicated, social pharmacy's methodologies and philosophies are drawn from the social and behavioural sciences and their selection is determined by the subject matter. For example, a political science approach would inform the relative influence that governments and pharmaceutical companies have on drug costs and on doctor's prescribing patterns. Indeed, in this way Greenwood (Chapter 13) examines the symbiotic relationship between the government and the pharmaceutical industry, and the bargaining tactics of each, revealing the complexities of policy making and the interplay between power and interests. A study of those who actually "consume" pharmaceutical products however, requires a different approach. For example, in a study of mothers' actions in response to their children's minor symptoms, and their use of pharmaceutical services, Cunningham-Burley (Chapter 6) employed a qualitative methodological approach involving interviews and health diaries. Interdisciplinarity is equally pertinent in the study of interprofessional relations. Harding *et al* (Chapter 5), also used a sociological approach to show how team work and relations between health care professionals is not something that occurs unproblematically. Indeed, professionals working closely together can often generate tensions and difficulties. Thus the analysis of the perceptions that members of the health care team have of each other is vital if we are to understand the nature of such difficulties – indeed this forms the nub of the chapter. An insight into what people think, and how they perceive situations, can only be gained by using qualitative methods.

Professionalisation

A profession is an occupational group which possesses certain characteristics, including a high level of technical expertise, a commitment to public service, monopoly of practice and autonomy over the content of its own work. They also have high prestige and status. Professionalisation, refers to the strategies which occupational groups pursue to attain and maintain professional status. The chapters by Aïach and Cèbe, Bottero, Britten and Harding *et al* are all informed by this sociological concept. Aïach and Cèbe (Chapter 2) describe how changes in the pharmacist's role have affected their job satisfaction. Pharmacists' satisfaction and status, traditionally derived from knowledge and skills required for drug preparation, have been undermined by the proliferation of pre-packaged drugs, such that pharmacists now look to other areas of work for satisfaction.

There has been a steady increase in the proportion of women entering the pharmaceutical profession. Bottero (Chapter 3) challenges the assumption that the increased proportion of woman pharmacists corresponds with a decline in the profession's status; indicating that in recent decades the status of the profession has increased. In this respect, she adds to current debates about the declining status of pharmacy which have tended to focus on issues such as the demise of skills in drug preparation to the exclusion of other more positive factors. She argues that pharmacists' enhanced status is evidenced by factors such as: degree level training; the higher qualifications required to enter schools of pharmacy; and entrants, who are increasingly likely to come from middle class backgrounds.

One new area of pharmacists' work relates to the development of computerised patient medication records (PMRs). Britten (Chapter 4), argues that PMRs have enhanced the professional status of pharmacists in relation to the medical profession. This is because PMRs provide access to information about patients hitherto denied to pharmacists and so, with this information, they are able to monitor the prescribing habits of doctors. PMRs also facilitate pharmacists' extended clinical role in that they are able to provide their clients with more informed advice.

As we discussed at the beginning of this chapter, an increasingly important aspect of all health professionals work is health education and health promotion. Health promotion, has been used as a vehicle by some professional groups, such as general medical practitioners to enhance their professional status.[11] Pharmacists are also playing a key role in health education and health promotion both in relation to specific health issues such as AIDS and drug misuse (see McKeganey and Barnard, Chapter 11 and Roberts and Harrison, Chapter 10) and to health more generally (see Smith, Chapter 7). The provision of a suitable environment to counsel clients is also discussed by Smith (Chapter 7) and by Blenkinsopp *et al* (Chapter 8).

Efficiency and Cost Effectiveness

There is a growing emphasis, in Western industrialised societies, on the effectiveness and efficiency of health care which has resulted, in part, from attempts to impose cost constraints. Governments are keen to contain the drugs bill, and doctors' prescribing patterns have consequently come under scrutiny. Davis (Chapter 12) provides an analysis of prescribing patterns in New Zealand and offers some reasons for apparent variations. Greenwood (Chapter 13) suggests that governments and the pharmaceutical industry are interdependent, though the pharmaceutical industry often holds the "strongest cards" in negotiations. However, through detailed analyses of key events such as the introduction of the "limited list" in the UK, he describes how an ability to wield political power is contingent on a given social and political context which is constantly changing.

Audit is another dimension of efficiency, with the activities of health workers being increasingly subject to surveillance to ensure that their services are cost-effective. The introduction of the internal market in the UK health service has led pharmacists to monitor and assess the efficacy of their work. Through the specification of the tasks conducted on wards by hospital pharmacists, Barber *et al* (Chapter 14) were able to provide a measurement of their duties which can be incorporated into contracts – the cornerstone of the internal market. As the authors point out, in a system which operates on market principles, it is essential that activities can be itemised so that they are not undersold or neglected.

Education and Communication

As pharmacists take on new roles and activities there have been commensurate developments in pharmacy education and training. Training in specific communication skills has become an integral element of pharmacy education. Being able to communicate with colleagues and/or clients requires specific skills and an awareness of others' circumstances. This involves a very different type of training to that required for the preparation of drugs. Hargie and Morrow (Chapter 9) provide both an insight into, and overview of, the types of communication skills relevant to pharmacy. Blenkinsopp *et al* (Chapter 8) on the other hand evaluate the effectiveness of pharmacist-client communication in the community.

Pharmacists are increasingly becoming problem solvers faced with a range of pragmatic queries – be they from mothers (Cunningham-Burley, Chapter 6) or other members of the health care team (Harding *et al*, Chapter 5) – for which they have to provide solutions. Reflecting these changes in practice, innovative changes have been made to pharmacy curricula in the UK (see Bates *et al*, Chapter 15) and Sweden (Bingerfors and Isacson, Chapter 16). These changes have involved the introduction of problem solving activities; students collaborating to generate solutions for themselves rather than being provided with detailed knowledge and information which they rote learn for examinations.

CONCLUSION

We have argued in this chapter that social pharmacy has emerged as a distinct field of study in response to wider social changes. These changes have seen the advent of new forms of health care which seek to promote health rather than simply treat disease and to provide an effective and efficient service to patients and clients. Innovations associated with these transformations have had significant effects on the daily activities of pharmacists. They are now spending more time communicating with clients, they are encouraged to work constructively with specific client groups, for example in needle-exchange schemes; they are having to monitor their workloads and they are prime users of new developments in information technology. Whilst these effects are, for the most part, beneficial they are not without difficulties. The identity of pharmacy is being recast and for the players involved this means that new skills have to be learned and the consequences of new activities have to be evaluated and assessed. The exploration of these issues is the very essence of social pharmacy.

REFERENCES

1. Harding G, Taylor KMG. Defining social pharmacy. *International Journal of Pharmacy Practice* 1993; 2: 62-63.
2. Bulmer M, Lewis J, Piachaud D. Social Policy: Subject or Object? In: Bulmer M, Lewis J, Piachaud D. eds. *The Goals of Social Policy.* London: Unwin Hyman; 1989.
3. Bunton R, Macdonald G. eds. *Health promotion: disciplines and diversity.* London: Routledge; 1992.
4. McKinlay JB. The promotion of health through planned sociopolitical change: challenges for research and policy. *Social Science and Medicine* 1993; 36: 109-117.
5. For example, McKeown T. *The Role of Medicine: Dream Mirage and Nemesis.* Oxford: Blackwell Scientific; 1979. Powels J. On the Limitations of Modern Medicine. *Science, Medicine and Man* 1973; 1: 1-30.
6. World Health Organisation. *Targets for Health for All.* Copenhagen: WHO Regional Office for Europe; 1985.
7. Lewis J. *What Price Community Medicine?* Brighton: Wheatsheaf; 1987.
8. Department of Health. *Health of the Nation.* London: HMSO (Cmd 1986); 1992.
9. Nuffield Committee of Inquiry into Pharmacy. *Pharmacy: A report to the Nuffield Foundation.* London: The Nuffield Foundation; 1986.
10. Turner BS. *Regulating Bodies: Essays in Medical Sociology.* London: Routledge; 1992, p.125.
11. Davis C. General Practitioners and the pull of prevention. *Sociology of Health and Illness* 1984: 6; 267-289.

CHAPTER TWO

PHARMACY IN CRISIS: THE CASE OF FRENCH PHARMACY

Pierre Aïach and Dominique Cèbe

INTRODUCTION

Before discussing what we believe to be the crisis in pharmacy and what pharmacists see as underlying this "crisis", we should explain our reasons for choosing this term. It is a term which is used frequently, and with various meanings, in the press and audio-visual media and in the scientific world. Edgar Morin, has observed that its widespread use has rendered it almost meaningless. Nevertheless he writes, "the word crisis serves to name the unnameable,"[1] and notes that the notion of crisis incorporates the idea of indecision. By this he means that crisis suggests that something is wrong and that things, which under normal circumstances are invisible, become apparent. He also notes that it refers to "the moment when, at the same time as disruption, uncertainties arise...". A time of crisis can therefore be the moment of truth, or conversely, a time of progression or regeneration. We have previously used the notion of crisis in this way in a book about serious illness and the ways in which it affects the lives of sick people and those close to them.[2] With respect to a profession, "crisis" can, according to Eliot Friedson[3], lead to a decline, which is evidenced by a loss of prestige and public confidence. It may involve the professionals becoming salaried employees which in turn may mean that they lose their independence (i.e. a qualified process of deprofessionalisation). Thus the professional no longer has the sole right or power to choose either the content of the work performed or the method of practice. In our current studies on the profession of pharmacy in France, we have sought to analyse the position of pharmacists in relation to their different interpretations of the notion of crisis.

Within a survey undertaken with community pharmacists, the term crisis was presented in such a way as to elicit either a positive or negative response. The pharmacists were asked the question: "Can we talk of a crisis in relation to the situation of the pharmacist in France today?" The notion of crisis which emerged from the pharmacists' responses corresponded to the financial and managerial dimensions of the concept. Another dimension which we expected to appear from the pharmacists' responses did not emerge in this survey, the notion of "identity crisis" which results from the hybrid nature of the pharmaceutical profession[4,5,6]: it is both highly scientific and also commercial as the pharmacist sells both medicines and so-called "para-pharmaceutical" products. In France the profession enjoys a monopoly of practice which is based on being awarded a university diploma after five years of study and provides the practitioner with a knowledge relating to the dispensing of medicines and prescribed and non-prescribed preparations.

The College of Pharmacy was created in Paris in 1777. The apothecaries in France succeeded in their struggle with doctors and various trade guilds which contested their independence in the preparation of medicines. Such preparations were frequently produced in accordance with very complex formulae. The production of master preparations, which was formerly the basis of the profession's creative and knowledgeable activity constituted, until the 1940s, the greater part of the pharmacist's work. However a considerable transformation occurred with the industrial production of medicines. The extremely rapid development of such proprietary products had the effect of considerably reducing the importance of compounding within pharmacies. In 1900, 90% of the pharmacist's activity consisted of the preparation of medicines, while in 1958 it was 30% and in 1966 just 17%.[7]

Given this change we might hypothesise that giving advice would come to form the primary basis for the pharmacist's quest for legitimacy and monopoly of practice. This hypothesis was tested in a sociological study published in 1978[8] which showed that although giving advice appeared to be by far and away the leading function identified by pharmacists, it represented only a small part of what they actually did. In fact selling products without giving advice to the purchaser constituted two thirds of their activity. Other studies, especially those conducted in the U.S.A., have yielded similar results. It would appear to be the case therefore, that offering of advice to clients is in fact far less important than is supposed or claimed by pharmacists themselves.[9,10]

Before undertaking our 1992 survey, we believed that since the above-mentioned study[8] was completed, developments within pharmacy could have only accentuated the division between the purely mercantile aspect of the pharmacist's activity and the social or public health dimension. In the latter, pharmacists both draw on their specialist knowledge and pursue altruistic activities such as advising patients, inspecting prescriptions and taking into account the patient's pathological profile. Pharmacists may well feel that they are confined by the straightjacket of increasingly numerous and interfering managerial regulations; that they are caught between a hypothetical aspiration to be useful and to justify (at least to themselves) their monopoly in the sale of medicines; that they are threatened by superstores trying to break into the market; and that they are under repeated attack by public bodies. Within this context pharmacists might feel ever more acutely a crisis of identity. This crisis could be traced back to the historical trauma produced by industrial medicine which has deprived the pharmacist's practice of the scientific and creative content enjoyed by his ancestor the apothecary. We will return to this point but first we will examine how pharmacists expressed their sense of crisis, their satisfaction with their chosen profession and their desire to continue to practice in it.

THE CRISIS AS IT IS LIVED

In 1992 we carried out a survey of community pharmacists practising in metropolitan France. Our postal questionnaire consisted of questions about their choice of profession, and their perceptions of their current and future functions. We present here those results which relate to the notion of crisis and in particular to those issues which concern the way pharmacists experience their professional practice and their relationship to their clients; their opinions about whether there is currently a "crisis" within pharmacy; their overall degree of satisfaction with the profession and its evolution over the past 20 years; their opinions about the future of the profession, trade unions, and government policy in relation to pharmacy; and what they perceive to be the main threats that they currently face.

The results presented here are taken from a representative sample of 340 pharmacists: 184 men (54%) and 156 women (46%). This distribution closely reflects the 1988 distribution of male and female pharmacists in France (respectively 57% and 43%). In our sample the pharmacists were slightly older (44 years old) than the 1988 average for France (41 years old).

THE EVOLUTION OF COMMUNITY PHARMACY IN FRANCE: 1970-1990

The way pharmacists perceived themselves was first and foremost as health care professionals (60%);[*] that is they prioritised their role as a health care adviser (cited by nearly 1 out of 2 pharmacists); their technical knowledge of medicines (1 in 3) or their role in checking prescriptions to assure the safety of clients (1 in 10). Following this, pharmacists saw themselves as managers or company heads (16%) who must deal with numerous administrative tasks. They also saw themselves as contact people, that is they felt that they fulfilled a social and

---

[*] For the majority of questions asked the pharmacists could give several different responses. The percentages given in the text are thus calculated based on the 340 pharmacists surveyed (% of PH) or more frequently, based on all the responses to one question (%)

humane role (16%). Finally, on a secondary level, they perceived themselves as shopkeepers specialising in dispensing medicine (4%).

This highly positive self-portrayal of the pharmacist's role, in particular placing great emphasis on the scientific and humane aspects of the profession rather than its more commercial dimension, is countered by their view of the evolution of the profession over the last two decades. In fact, two thirds of the responses emphasised negative aspects of this evolution. Above all, they mentioned a sharp increase in the amount of paperwork (1 pharmacist in 2); the disappearance, or the diminution, of the creative side to their work (master preparations in particular) (1 pharmacist in 5); and the decrease in profits (13% of PH). Responses highlighting positive aspects of the evolution were in the minority (10%). These basically referred to the acquisition of more specialised scientific knowledge because of the existence of new drug entities.

This highly critical judgement of the evolution of the profession highlights the somewhat theoretical and idealised conception that pharmacists have of their own role. This conception is the synthesis of the high esteem they hold for their role and the reality of what their practice is like.

JOB SATISFACTION AMONG COMMUNITY PHARMACISTS

When questioned about the satisfaction their profession afforded them, pharmacists mentioned first of all the contact they have with clients (26%) and their social role (16%). Next they mentioned the scientific and medical side of practice (13%) and the gratitude expressed by their clients (11%). Other factors were mentioned by only a small number, for example some referred to the independence the profession allows them (8%); the material rewards such as job security and a comfortable income (6%), and finally the diversity and active quality of their profession (6%).

Less than 10% of pharmacists surveyed derived no satisfaction, very little, or less and less satisfaction from their jobs. We could emphasise here that the satisfaction derived from specific aspects of their work: giving advice, scientific knowledge, working in health care etc., is decidedly less than what one could associate with any commercial activity: contact with other people, client fidelity, independence, profits, even if one considers that the social role is connected to the specific professional side of being a pharmacist.

When questioned about the reasons behind their dissatisfaction, pharmacists especially mentioned the administrative tasks they must perform and the heavy amount of paperwork involved (28%); the hostility shown by public authorities and the feeling of dependence towards the government (18%); and financial difficulties (14%). The decrease in the scientific content of practice was relatively unimportant (7%), as was the difficulty of the job (6%), problems with the clientele (6%), and the pharmacist's deteriorating image (5%).

Even before the notion of crisis was introduced it was evident that pharmacists were extremely unhappy with public authorities which implemented numerous measures that diminished their profits, as well as with the existence of certain constraints such as the "tiers-payant" system* that creates cash difficulties and, most importantly, obliges them to perform tedious and time-consuming administrative tasks.

Does satisfaction in the end prevail over dissatisfaction? One could think so in view of the answers given to the question about satisfaction with the choice of profession. Two thirds of pharmacists gave a positive response and the remaining third was split equally between negative responses and mixed feelings. This contentment nonetheless seems somewhat tempered when one asks if they would make the same choice of profession today: only 46% said yes, while 40% would not.

This relative divergence of opinion can probably be explained by the fact that the two questions do not refer to the same reality. The first is largely concerned with the professional past, when pharmacists may have experienced more prosperous times, while the second question essentially refers to their current situation and all the problems associated with it. Opinions are further tempered when it comes to the question of whether or not the pharmacists questioned would encourage their children to choose the same profession. Nearly 1 out of 2 would advise neither a son nor daughter to make this choice, while those who would encourage it were a mere 16%. This can be interpreted as a sign of a pessimistic vision of the profession's future.

PHARMACY IN CRISIS?

In relation to the current state of pharmacy, 85% of the pharmacists thought that one could indeed speak in terms of a crisis. The responsibility for this crisis they overwhelmingly attributed to public authorities, with only 1 in 10 admitting that responsibility could be shared among the authorities, trades unions, and the profession.

For one quarter of the pharmacists the crisis began before 1982; for another quarter between 1982 and 1988; for a third quarter in 1988, when the "taux de marque" (profit margin) was lowered; and for the remainder after 1988, notably

---

* With this system, increasingly in use, the pharmacist advances the proportion of cost that will be reimbursed by Social Security and sends to Social Security the forms that allow him to be repaid.

in 1990, when the M.D.L. was established and the S.H.P. abolished.* For these pharmacists the crisis is primarily of a financial order (55%) for several reasons: because of various measures enacted by public authorities that go counter to their interests (profit margin, M.D.L., S.H.P.); the fact that certain medicines and preparations are no longer reimbursed by Social Security; cash difficulties because of delays in being repaid by Social Security in the case of the "tiers-payant" system; an increase in taxes and social charges; and intransigence on the part of banks and rising prices for those who recently acquired a pharmacy.

Other responses concerned problems of competition (particularly with superstores), the tendency towards commercialisation (10%), and the problems of financing Social Security due to an overconsumption of medicine. They see this as tied to the popularisation of medicine and people's irresponsibility (9%). Less than 1 pharmacist in 20 mentioned a reason related to the "professional identity crisis" discussed previously. However this does not necessarily mean that the pharmacists surveyed do not feel deeply this "structural crisis", rather when faced with the term crisis their spontaneous reaction is to speak of whatever is posing problems for them at the moment and this is most likely to be the difficulties they face daily, which exist because of an evolution by which they are heavily penalised and, in spite of themselves, transformed into an instrument of political power trying to cut back on health care expenses.

Thus, what they declare to be the "major problems they must deal with" are above all financial (48%), administrative and managerial (20%). Far less important are problems connected to working conditions (10%), personnel (6%), keeping their knowledge up to date and developing their advice-giving function (6%).

HOW WILL THE CRISIS BE RESOLVED?

One pharmacist in 5 has a dark vision of the future and sees no possible resolution, or at least none in the immediate future, judging that the situation can only get worse. Given the way pharmacists characterise the crisis, they logically expect its resolution to come primarily from public authorities (41%), whether this be through a change in government or policy changes. These might involve the suppression or readjustment of measures relating to them; confirmation of their monopoly and the "numerus clausus" (currently one pharmacy for 2000 to

---

* M.D.L.: "Marge Dégressive Lissée": profit decreases as the price of the medicine increases.

S.H.P.:"Supplément Honoraires Pharmaceutiques": Responsibility tax of 0.40% collected for keeping an "ordonnancier." This is a register where the pharmacist records the name of the products prescribed containing "poisonous substances," as well as the name of the prescribing doctor and the name and address of the patient

3000 inhabitants, depending upon its location); dialogue with the profession; the abandonment of hostile attitudes; and finally, measures affecting the way Social Security functions. Very few pharmacists foresee a possible resolution through initiatives coming from the profession (8%), although they feel it would be beneficial to rehabilitate both the image and the role of the pharmacist.

WHAT DO PHARMACISTS PLAN ON DOING?

While a quarter of pharmacists did not envisage taking any particular steps in the near future, the remainder did. Some considered reducing expenses either by making personnel changes through lay-offs or hiring less qualified personnel (22%), or by improving the management of the pharmacy, notably reducing costs and managing their stock more sensibly (16%). Others planned to try to increase turnover by adopting a more "aggressive" commercial stance, particularly with regard to para-pharmaceutical products. The most discouraged pharmacists saw a drastic solution as the only way out: selling the pharmacy without plans to purchase another (10%).

THE FUTURE OF PHARMACY

Pharmacists do not foresee a particularly rosy future, considering the numerous threats they face. These threats take various forms but essentially originate in the policy adopted or envisaged by public authorities. In fact, nearly 6 pharmacists in 10 thought the authorities desired that pharmacy in its present form should disappear altogether. They gave various possible reasons for this: so that they might control the profession and the dispensing of medicines (14%); to favour superstores and big businesses over small pharmacies (17%); to reduce health care costs and make sure that the pharmacist does not get unduly rich at the expense of Social Security (28%); or finally, because of political ideology or demagogy, which at times goes hand in hand with incompetence and a will to destroy (25%).

THREATS TO THE FUTURE OF COMMUNITY PHARMACY IN FRANCE

The disappearance of small pharmacies, especially in rural areas was perceived as a major threat (15%). These pharmacies have already been affected by cash difficulties and the fact that their turnover depends heavily on the sale of medicines. They are also the pharmacies most penalised by measures affecting profit margins, especially the M.D.L. system. It disadvantages them because a large part of their clientele is made up of chronically ill, aged patients who purchase expensive prescribed medications. Closely linked to this is the threat of impoverishment of all pharmacies, whose profitability is progressively decreasing (13%).

The second kind of threat is competition (16%), which can manifest itself in the form of "unfair" competition such as from pharmacists who practice in shopping centres. When questioned on this point a majority of pharmacists (71%) declared themselves to be against such an arrangement, arguing that it not only represents unfair competition and a diversion of clients from fellow pharmacists practising in less favourable locations, but also means exercising an essentially commercial activity, to the detriment of the pharmacist's advice-giving function. This competition could also take a legal form. It would consist of eliminating the "numerus clausus" or giving up the monopoly on certain products such as vitamin C, to the benefit of superstores. In response to a question about the sale of health care products in superstores, 9 pharmacists out of 10 expressed their disapproval, highlighting the potential dangers, whether it be for the clients' sake, since so-called health care products, which they consider to be like medicines, are not harmless, or for the pharmacists' sake. For them the sale of borderline health care products in superstores constitutes a breach of their monopoly, a breach which could grow until it touched the sale of medicines proper.

It is clear that the loss of the monopoly on the sale of medicines would mean the demise of the practising pharmacist as such and thus it is essential for him/her that this monopoly has recognised legitimacy. This legitimacy seems to be contested, especially by consumer protection associations that have conducted investigations showing grave failings both in terms of advice and the inspection of products supplied according to a prescription.[11,12]

When pharmacists were questioned about whether or not their monopoly is justified, they were quick to emphasise their specific knowledge of medicine, which they considered to be indispensable to understanding the potency of drugs and for the advice required upon dispensing (58%). Some mentioned the scientific knowledge they have acquired (15%) and their availability (9%), especially for advice; others, the overconsumption of medicine they help to avoid (5%) and the guarantee they offer in terms of professional regulation and professional ethics (4%). Still others mentioned the fact that they know their clients and are familiar with their therapy (3.5%).

Despite the emphasis pharmacists place on their familiarity with medicine and the verification that should take place upon its dispensing, in particular to watch for drug interactions, they acknowledge that certain shortcomings are possible on this point. In fact, when questioned about incidents of prescriptions not being verified as revealed in investigations conducted by "Que Choisir"[11] and "L'impatient"[12] nearly 4 pharmacists in 10 judged this "plausible" or "possible in certain cases." They attributed it to poor working conditions (17%), a lack of training (8%) and the maxim "errare humanum est" (8%). On the other hand, they were much more critical of these same investigations for their conclusions regarding the giving of advice; among the 52% that had heard about the investigations, two thirds found them "tendentious," "nonrepresentative," and the fruit of "scandal press," while 1 in 5 thought there was some truth to what they said, and that this should push pharmacists to do better.

The pharmacists' rather lively reaction to the subject of their shortcomings in the area of advice can be explained at least in part by the importance they place on advice, if only on a symbolic level, as a factor lending legitimacy to their existence.[8] In fact, 8 pharmacists in 10 placed great importance on advice in their practice, 6 of them going so far as to say it was of "primordial," "fundamental," or of "enormous importance".

Nevertheless, for two thirds of pharmacists their giving of advice was not, practically speaking, as important as they would like it to be, due to certain obstacles that confronted them. For instance, a lack of time and availability due especially to the burden of administrative work (40%), the fact that clients, often in a hurry or knowing exactly what they want, do not solicit their advice (30%) and a lack of competent personnel (8%). Very few (5%) challenged their own knowledge or mentioned the prohibition to dispense medication other than what is specifically prescribed (5%).

In spite of all these obstacles, more than half the pharmacists (52%) estimate that for every 10 clients coming into the pharmacy, 6 to 10 "receive some advice of one kind or another." This may be an overestimation when compared to the results of other studies.[6,9]

The third type of threat to pharmacy (13%) concerns the pharmacist's loss of independence because of the government's growing interference and the possibility that "chains" of pharmacies or large distributors could control the profession. In the eyes of some pharmacists this possibility could be favoured by the opening of the European Market. Nonetheless the European Community does not seem to pose a threat for pharmacies, even if 1 in 5 pharmacists is worried to some degree about the opening up of the "European Market"; it is seen as potentially a good thing for 7% of them, or as likely to bring few changes for 11%. Yet numerous pharmacists (41%) declared themselves incapable of responding to this question either due to a lack of information or because they considered it too difficult to assess the possible effects at that time.

In the face of all these threats to the pharmaceutical profession, present or future, real or hypothetical, the action of trade unions is judged "insufficient," "poorly adapted," or even "nonexistent" by the great majority of pharmacists (80%). A mere 15% judged it "satisfactory." However, 70% of them said they belonged to a union and, among this 70%, 11% have some sort of responsibility within the union.

As stated previously, the pharmacy crisis, defined from the responses given by the pharmacists surveyed is essentially financial in nature, while any reference to elements that could be linked to the notion of an identity crisis is almost completely absent. One can, of course, put forward the explanation already mentioned, of preeminent importance being accorded to the more acute problems pharmacists meet in their daily practice. The measures concerning pharmacists, enacted in recent years and having contributed significantly to the financial crisis, can perhaps account for the non-confirmation of the hypothesis we formulated of an intensification of the "structural" crisis in relation to the evolution of an increasingly commercialised pharmacy. In fact this hypothesis seems to be confirmed neither in the responses directly concerning the crisis nor in those related to the "contradiction between the commercial function and the functions of advising, verifying, and educating," a contradiction that the pharmacists for the most part do not perceive. They do not consider these functions to be opposed because of the existence of rules of ethics that they feel bound to respect, or because of the nature of this contradiction, as certain authors have suggested.[4]

Another possible reason the pharmacists' remarks made no reference to an identity crisis could be the positive changes in attitude that certain pharmacists, notably young ones, seem to display towards the role of company head, in relation to transformations in the social world (less stigmatisation of material success). There is also less difference between the way they see the profession at the moment they chose it and the reality of what pharmacy is really like as a commercial enterprise.

What will be the consequences of the financial crisis that pharmacists complain about, aggravated by a steadily increasing stream of paperwork? In a pessimistic vision of the future one can imagine pharmacists caught up in a current that could carry them to their ruin: watching profits erode, obliged to become increasingly commercial in order to survive, crushed under the weight of administrative tasks, obliged to work with fewer and less qualified employees, with the time devoted to giving advice and inspecting prescriptions dramatically decreased. In this case the challenge to the legitimacy of pharmacists' monopoly on the supply of medicines would be fully warranted. This is, of course, a "worst case scenario." It is highly unlikely that it will come about, especially given the new political context in France, even though some pharmacists surveyed envisaged it. The fact remains nonetheless, that the situation of pharmacy, already in difficulty financially, is weakened by the challenge, at times virulent, to the foundations of its monopoly. This is a challenge to its very existence, which is based on giving advice and checking prescriptions. If pharmacists do not fulfil, or fulfil poorly, these functions, which legitimise the existence of a sales monopoly that other merchants do not have, what else will they be able to base their monopoly on? Certain authors have suggested possible ways out, and a form of reprofessionalisation in the development of clinical pharmacy.[13,14] However, in the French context clinical pharmacy is only at the embryonic stage and its implementation would pose serious problems, if only in its relationship with the medical profession.

However, even if one considers that the criticisms against them are to a certain degree founded, pharmacists in France are located in neighbourhoods and provide a service that is generally carried out with efficiency, competence and availability.

ACKNOWLEDGEMENT

This study received financial assistance from Giphar-France Association of Pharmacists.

REFERENCES

1. Morin E. *Sociologie*. Paris: Fayard; 1984.
2. Aïach P, Kaufmann A, Waissman R. *Vivre une maladie grave*. Paris: Meridiens Klincksieck; 1989.
3. Friedson E. *Professional Powers, a study of the institutionalisation of formal knowledge*. Chicago: Chicago University Press; 1986.
4. Chappell NL, Barnes GE. Professional and business role orientations among practising pharmacists. *Social Science and Medicine* 1984; 18: 103-110.
5. Holloway SWF, Jewson ND, Mason DJ. Reprofessionalisation or occupational imperialism? Some reflections on pharmacy in Britain. *Social Science and Medicine* 1986; 23: 323-332.
6. Aïach P. Une profession conflictuelle: la pharmacie d'officine. In: Aïach P, Fassin D. eds. *Sociologie des professions de santé*. Paris: Editions de l'Espace Europeen; 1992.
7. Fabre R, Dillman G. *Histoire de la pharmacie*. Paris: Que sais-je? Presses Universitaires de France; 1963.
8. Aïach P. *Les pharmaciens d'officine: contradictions et ambiguïté d'une profession singulière*. Thesis in Sociology. Paris X: Nanterre; 1978.
9. Roney J, Nall M. *Medication practices in a community, an exploratory study*. Menlo Park, CA: Stanford Research Institute; 1966.
10. Watkins RL, Norwood GJ. Pharmacist drug consultation behaviour. *Social Science and Medicine* 1978; 12: 235-239.
11. Bert C. Peut-on se fier aux pharmaciens? *Que Choisir Santé* 1990; 3: 8-13.
12. Marescot B. 100 pharmaciens au banc d'essai. Et mauvais conseillers en plus. *L'Impatient* 1990; 135: 18-20.
13. Bardeley D. Une opportunité. *Prescrire* 1989; 4: 35-36.
14. Birenbaum A. Reprofessionalisation in pharmacy. *Social Science and Medicine* 1982; 16: 871-878.

CHAPTER THREE

THE CHANGING FACE OF PHARMACY?

Gender and explanations of women's entry to pharmacy

Wendy Bottero

INTRODUCTION

This chapter looks at the changing identity of pharmacists. It argues that processes of change in pharmacy represent a challenge to theories of employment which must be addressed if those theories are to have any explanatory value. Commentators within the profession and from the social sciences have noted the increasing number of women entering pharmacy, but there has been a failure to locate this within wider processes of change. Sociological theories which attempt to explain women's professional careers have stressed gender divisions in employment, arguing that women have only gained entry as jobs have declined in pay and prestige. When patterns of female entry to pharmacy are examined in some detail, however, it becomes apparent that, although linked to a re-structuring of employment opportunities within the profession, the changing identity of pharmacists is a more complex process than most theories have suggested. The object of this chapter is to question whether it is helpful to see women's position within the professions in terms of gender disadvantage.

Patterns of entry and employment in pharmacy indicate that women's entry is a part of general processes of re-structuring which are transforming the identity and employment of all pharmacists. The concentration on gender divisions which has characterised sociological accounts of pharmacy has resulted in the neglect of other important variations and in the under-estimation of the extent of change. A re-examination of theoretical categories is necessary if the developments in pharmacy are to be fully understood. In the following section I will look at the way in which sociological theory explains women's employment in the professions, and attempt to demonstrate some of the problems of such accounts. While the description of women in male-dominated professions as "gender subordination" is initially plausible it is inadequate.

GENDER AND MALE-DOMINATED PROFESSIONS

The concentration of women in low paid and disadvantaged employment has been extensively documented. In privileged jobs, women are more noted for their absence or, where they are to be found, for their marginalisation. A division between female-dominated "semi-professions" and male-dominated "professions" has long been accepted. However in the 1970s and 1980s there has been an increase in women entering male-dominated professions such as, medicine, law, accountancy and banking, in both Britain and the United States.[1,2] Explanations which focused on women's exclusion now have to deal with women's presence. With some notable exceptions, the conclusions have been pessimistic, with authors questioning the privilege of women's professional jobs. The entry of women has variously been described as a "hollow victory", a "disheartening paradox" and a "contradictory process", and it has been suggested that women are in the professions "in name only".

American literature is particularly cynical about whether female entry to male-dominated professions constitutes "progress". Even when authors do point to real changes their approach is in terms of issues of gender segregation and subordination. There is the repeated observation that within professions, women tend to work apart from men, in jobs which have lower pay and prestige. They argue that this pattern of working represents the "gendering" of employment structure into "men's work" and "women's work". So, for example, leading British commentators Crompton and Sanderson, declare themselves "cautiously optimistic" about the prospects of women breaking down sex segregation at work[3]. But their analysis depends on questioning whether changes in women's employment situation affects "gendered" patterns of working. So whilst an overall increase in women gaining qualifications has allowed women to enter male-dominated professions, Crompton and Sanderson[2] divide such qualifications and occupations by the likely career paths they give rise to. They suggest that women who have entered professions with more flexible working arrangements – such as pharmacy – have had discontinuous careers, with breaks and periods in part-time work which, they argue, represents the old pattern of distinctive styles of "women's work". In such professions, therefore, women have entered 'without giving rise to any major transformation of gender relationships'.[3]

A common theme is the description of female employment in male-dominated professions as "continuity in change". Whilst women have entered new employment areas differences between male and female professionals are still observed. Several processes are identified. Firstly the channelling of women into relatively less desirable sectors of the professions, for example, lower status specialisms, and their over-representation at the bottom of career hierarchies and in part-time work. The emergence of "gender-typing" has also been pointed out, with women being allocated to jobs "appropriate" to their gender. So the construction of jobs as being "caring" or requiring a "female touch" has been seen as part of women's direction into "women's work". It is argued that while women may have gained entry to male bastions they have not done so on the same terms as men, so their presence does not represent any breakdown in gender segregation or women's employment disadvantage. Kaufman has questioned whether women in male-dominated occupations are "professionals" in quite the same way as their male peers, since,

> '...most find themselves located in subsidiary positions within prestige
> professions or in positions that do not accord them the autonomy, prestige,
> or pay customarily associated with the professional image.'[4]

It has also been suggested, mainly by American authors, that there are a growing number of "secondary" jobs within the professions. This is a model of the professions segmenting into privileged and secondary sectors, with the development of secondary employment part of the process of female entry. For example, Carter and Carter argue that there is a growing split between prestige jobs with good pay and autonomy and a new sector of fragmented and routinized jobs.

It is this latter sector, they argue, that most women are entering, and that, '...this routinization has played a large role in removing barriers to women's professional employment'.*

This form of analysis suggests that women's gains are more apparent than real, for example, as Sokoloff argues:

> 'More women enter these professions just as they are changing – to be less
> under the control of the professionals themselves, less powerful, less
> profitable, and less prestigious.'[5]

Both description and explanation in such accounts use the categories of gender divisions. Differences between women and men are described as gender segregation, and the development of such patterns in male-dominated professions is seen as the same process of women's subordination which can be observed in less privileged areas of women's employment. Women

---

* Economists and sociologists suggest that national labour markets are segmented into different labour markets sectors. So, for example, dual labour market theory argues that there is a division between a primary sector, which is made up of highly paid jobs which offer clear career structures, and a secondary sector which comprises low paid jobs which offer little in the way of advancement, acquisition of skills or secure employment.

professionals are generally found in relatively lower status jobs and this is said to reflect women's overall lower status and power in society in that; '...what have been labelled gains for women reflect the elaboration of a sexual division of labour *within* detailed occupations that were predominantly male in the past.'[6] The problem with the literature on women's entry to male-dominated professions is that by stressing continuity, and focusing on gender differences, the complexity and specificity of women's employment situation tends to be lost. Ironically, in a literature dominated by case-studies, there has been a level of theoretical abstraction and generalisation about the processes of entry and description of employment patterns which is misleading. Because female professional "specialisms" are of relatively lower status women's subordinate status in society is seen as decisive in their allocation to them.

Female employment in male-dominated professions is therefore seen as a particular instance of a more general structure of women's disadvantage at work. However, pointing to continuities of employment between professional and non-professional women does not adequately describe the position of women in male-dominated professions or explain their presence there. The argument used to be that women were excluded from the professions because they were privileged forms of employment. Now that women are increasing in numbers it is their relative disadvantage rather than their privilege which is accentuated. However, even if relatively disadvantaged, these women are now in well paid, high status positions from which they were formerly excluded.

Arguments of a developing professional secondary labour market can be seen as an attempt to address the issue of increasing female entry but again there is a tendency to minimise the extent to which real change has occurred. Women's presence is explained by the decline in rewards in male-dominated professions, which implies that their jobs are not really privileged. Carter and Carter's[1] position on new areas of women's professional employment is that:

'Although they require a fair amount of formal schooling, a large number of these jobs have become low-paying, routine, and dead-end – much like other occupations employing large numbers of women.'

This comparison draws together individuals in widely differing circumstances, so that gender categories become extremely generalised.

It is true to say that authors have acknowledged variations in women's employment, and are not unaware of the privilege inherent in women's jobs in the professions. However, these factors remain incidental to theoretical explanations because the thrust of accounts is to use categories of gender segregation and subordination. It is important to draw a distinction between low status jobs and jobs that are merely of *lower* status, because the divisions between professional and non-professional women are arguably at least as great as those between women and men within the professions. There are important differences between women's and men's professional employment, but to see women's entry as a process of continuing subordination is to adopt the most generalised of explanations. There may well be "continuity in change" but explanations must be able to account for both, change as well as continuity, in a coherent and integrated fashion.

Part of the difficulty with explaining the change lies in the fact that any discussions of change tend to be hijacked by discussions of "progress". The argument is that because professional women are segregated in apparently the same fashion as women in less privileged jobs there is no challenge to the gender order and therefore no real progress. Progress is apparently only possible if non-gendered patterns of working emerge. But since the identification of gendered patterns rests on sex differences it is clear that considerable change in women's employment patterns can occur without it being "progress", since aggregate differences may remain. The focus of attention on whether female entry to male-dominated professions represents a challenge to gender segregation has distracted attention from the broader question of how it has challenged *theories* of gender segregation. Thus there is an increasing gulf between theory and the patterns and processes that theory addresses. As we shall see in accounts of pharmacy, the meaning of developments within the professions can only be captured by a much wider analysis.

PATTERNS OF ENTRY AND EMPLOYMENT IN PHARMACY

Women have been a majority of entrants to UK pharmacy since the late 1960s and so a substantial number of them are relatively well advanced in their careers. The process of entry can therefore be examined in some detail. The profession of pharmacy has been used by several authors to examine processes of feminisation, for instance; Crompton and Sanderson[2,3] in the UK and Reskin and Roos[6] in the USA.

Crompton and Sanderson see employment patterns in pharmacy as an example of the gendered division of labour: female entry associated with the development of "feminised niches" for women. They describe women's distribution between the two major sectors of pharmacy – the hospital service and community pharmacy – as both vertical and horizontal segregation. Women are over-represented in the hospital service where they predominate (64%), reflecting the "caring" interpersonal image of that sector and the lower rates of pay. Community pharmacy by contrast, with its long hours, entrepreneurial image and higher pay, is male-dominated (65%). Although the proportion of women have increased in community pharmacy, this mirrors the increase in part-time work in the community sector. Because of the wide availability of part-time work in pharmacy, Crompton and Sanderson[3] argue that women are able to combine home and work commitments and, in the context of rising qualification levels for all women, it is this which explains female entry. Their understanding of increased female entry into pharmacy is that it has occurred without disruption to conventional gender divisions of labour. Despite observing the convergence of male and female working patterns with, for example, more women working full-time and men part-time, the combination of domestic and work commitments that pharmacy permits serves to '...reproduce the gender order as a whole, in that women are subordinate to men.'[3]

Reskin and Roos[6], writing about US pharmacy, see feminisation in the context of increasing secondary employment, with both the technical job content and employment prospects of the pharmacist having been degraded. In other words, women increase participation as rewards and opportunities worsen. Reskin and Roos see this as the operation of gender hierarchy with women in subordinate positions which men no longer wish to work in. Indeed, in the post-war years in both the US and UK large manufacturers have taken over the compounding of drugs, introducing pre-packaged unit-dose preparations. Reskin and Roos argue this has "clericalised" the pharmacist's job, reducing it to dispensing and record-keeping. They also point to the growth in large chain store pharmacies, and the reduction of independent ownership, as evidence of declining opportunities. They say that the functions of pharmacists employed by chain stores, '...increasingly resemble those of retail sales clerks, a low status, traditionally female occupation'

Arguments of de-skilling and segmentation have been made in the US on the basis of observed change. Aspects of similar change have occurred in the UK – such as the increasing importance of chain stores and use of pre-packed drugs – and do seem to be related to female entry. However, de-skilling and segmentation is not a helpful explanation of UK patterns. We should be careful of seeing jobs as secondary just because women are in them. The period of supposed 'de-skilling' in pharmacy has also been a period of increasing professionalisation. In the UK the Royal Pharmaceutical Society's policy has been to attempt to dispel the "trade" image of the work and to present the job as the delivery of a professional service rather than the sale of medicines by a shopkeeper. Training has increased in length and changed from an apprenticeship to a degree only qualification. Within hospitals specialisms such as clinical pharmacy have developed with pharmacists taking an advisory role in the ward team (see Barber et al, this volume). Budgets for "practice research" have greatly increased and the academic nature of pharmacy has been strengthened. Pharmacists have therefore resisted de-skilling and most crucially, have maintained their monopoly on the dispensing of potentially dangerous drugs.

Any comparison of pharmacists to sales clerks, therefore, misses the influence of professional standing on employment position. Women pharmacists work alongside technicians and sales assistants, who are usually female, and often perform similar tasks. However, by virtue of their professional standing women pharmacists are in an infinitely more advantaged employment situation, with greater pay, status and control over their working environment than the women they work alongside. To draw a comparison between low status female workers and female pharmacists who are of lower status than their male peers, on the grounds that as women they share a common employment situation is to stretch gender categories very far.

However, it is true to say that there has been a substantial re-structuring of opportunities in pharmacy over the period of female entry. Crompton and Sanderson point to an increase in part-time work,[2,3] but this must be seen as part of a more general re-structuring of employment. Most of the increase in part-time work has occurred in the community sector, which has also seen a decline in full-time working. So part-time employment has increased in actual numbers and in relative importance. At the same time there has been a steady fall in the number of pharmacies since 1955, from around 15,000 to just over 11,000. Chain store pharmacies have increased in importance whilst independent ownership has been squeezed. The career consequences of these changes are that employee and part-time posts have increased at the expense of ownership, which has traditionally been regarded as better paid and the destination of most older men. So the emergence of part-time working is part of larger scale re-organisations where structured career development over the life course has been replaced by more marginal posts for the young, the part-time and the semi-retired. For Reskins and Roos[6] in the US, this represents gender subordination because women are channelled into lower status positions and their numbers increase as overall prospects worsen. However, if we look in some detail at the UK pattern of entry and how it relates to re-structuring it becomes apparent that the relationship between worsening prospects and female entry is mediated by the raising of educational requirements for the profession, and this *up-grading* has a direct correspondence with rising female numbers.

The Royal Pharmaceutical Society's professionalisation policy has raised academic standards of entry. Up until 1948 pharmacists qualified by taking a 3–5 year articled apprenticeship, followed by a 1 year academic course. In the 1950s–60s the college component was increased to 2 and then 3 years, and the apprenticeship replaced by a year of post-graduate training. After 1967 pharmacy became a degree course only. So entrance requirements have been raised, the length of study increased, and the standing of the professional qualification improved precisely over the period of female entry. Figure 1 shows the percentage of women in schools of pharmacy from 1962–87. The move to degree status would have started to take effect around 1968–9 and it is apparent that the biggest percentage jump – of 10% – occurs in the years 1969–71. The

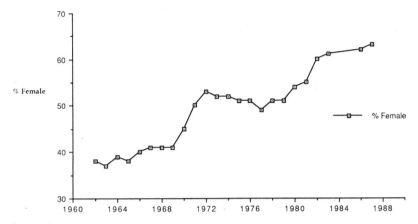

Source: Calculated from data supplied by The Royal Pharmaceutical Society of Great Britain

Figure 1: Percentage Female in U.K. Schools of Pharmacy: 1962–87
(Home students only)

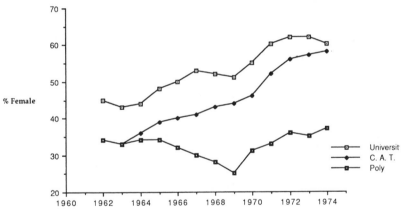

Source: Calculated from data in *The Pharmaceutical Journal* relevant years and from data
supplied by The Royal Pharmaceutical Society of Great Britain

Figure 2: Percentage Female at Schools of Pharmacy by Institution: 1962–1974
(Home Students Only)

second peak in the late 1970s is probably due to cuts in teacher training places
which Crompton and Sanderson[3] argue had a knock-on effect on female entry
to the professions. The rise in the status of the qualification appears to have a
positive relationship with female numbers.

A similar effect can be observed looking at the relationship between status of
qualifying institution and female numbers. Figure 2 shows the percentage of
women pharmacy students at three types of institutions: universities, colleges
of advanced technology and polytechnics between 1962–74. This shows that

women's share has always been greater in the higher status institutions. The shift upwards in female representation after 1967 – the move to degree status – shows up very clearly in all 3 lines. The middle line shows female representation at colleges of advanced technology, which achieved university status in 1966. Again, with the rise in the institutions' status the female proportion increases.

The entry of women is consistently associated with increases in the status of the professional qualification and with the attempts by the Pharmaceutical Society to professionalise the pharmacist's role. This could be interpreted as evidence that women competing with men have to be better simply to gain admission, and women applicants are thought to be better qualified. Yet it is difficult to describe as "subordination" a situation where women get directed to more prestigious institutions and increase in numbers with the status of the training. This is not to suggest that professionalisation has "caused" the entry of women, but it does mean that secondary professional employment cannot be seen as an adequate explanation. The process of entry cannot be associated with a decline in professional standing, the process is much more complex, as it is the interplay between professionalisation and re-structuring which produces the pattern of entry that we have seen.

On closer examination it becomes apparent that up-grading has not just had consequences for female numbers, and that "feminisation" is perhaps an inadequate description of the processes occurring in pharmacy. There have also been changes in the identity of male entrants to the profession. Looking at a small sample of pharmacists in Edinburgh it is possible to examine the class origins of entrants over time. There are a number of things to bear in mind however. Firstly, Scotland is rather different from the overall UK picture in that the proportion of women in pharmacy is higher. The percentage in Edinburgh is over 60% female whilst in the UK it stands at just over 40%. The pattern of entry in Scotland is almost identical to the pattern of entry in England, but starts rather earlier, and from a higher base line. Secondly, in looking at changes over time, registration cohorts have been used, but these represent "survivors" on the register of pharmacists, so caution should be used in interpreting the data, since this may not represent successive cohorts that started out in pharmacy.

Table 1 shows the class origins of succeeding registration "survivor" cohorts. In looking at stratification position the Cambridge Scale of Occupations was used. This is a continuous measure of occupations in terms of similarity of lifestyle and therefore of generalised advantage/disadvantage, the higher the score the higher the social origin[7]. The Table groups women and men by the year of registration and shows, for each group, the mean scale score for parental occupation. Parental occupation was taken at the time of the respondent's leaving school. If both parents were in paid employment the highest scoring job was used.

This Table shows that on average women pharmacists are of higher social

TABLE 1: Class Level by Sex and Registration Year (Edinburgh Sample)

	Parental Occupation			
YEAR REGISTERED	MALES	FEMALES	TOTAL	MALE % OF COHORT
TO 1949	40.67	61.75	47.13 (n=45)	68
1950–59	54.95	52.64	53.70 (n=22)	46
1960–69	64.87	61.70	62.67 (n=36)	30
1970–79	51.82	61.99	57.81 (n=56)	42
1980–89	58.22	62.29	61.10 (n=89)	28
Total	51.78	61.26	57.39 (n=89)	
	F Value	P	(missing 25)	
Males	3.68	0.01		
Females	0.48	Not Significant		

(Mean Cambridge Scale Score)

origins than men. There have also been important changes over time. Overall there has been a net increase in class origins, reaching a peak in the 1960s and with a slight fluctuation in the 1970s. Looking at gender breakdowns over time we can see that, with some fluctuation, women's class origins have stayed the same. The most change has occurred in male class, which rises sharply, after 1949, to reach a peak in the 1960s when it falls somewhat, but still to a higher level than it started. Using one-way analysis of variance the difference in mean class level across the year groups is statistically significant for men, but not for women. As we have already seen the educational up-grading started after 1948, with most of the changes occurring in the 1950s and 60s, culminating in degree status in 1967. The timing of these changes in male class origin is therefore significant, occurring at exactly the point of status changes.

Even more significantly the class composition of males seems to vary with the proportion of males in the cohort. The higher the stratification score of the males in the cohort the fewer the men there are. When the score falls in the 1970s the male proportion recovers, only to fall again when the mean score increases in the 1980s. There has been an expansion in service class occupations (that is personal and business services in both the public and private sector) throughout the UK postwar, and Table 1 will reflect these changes. However, in Table 1 it is only male class that rises, and when, contrary to national trends, male class falls in the 1970s, the relationship with male numbers in the cohort still holds. According to the Edinburgh data, there does seem to be a direct correspondence between status changes in the qualification, and the class and number of male entrants to the profession. Male social class rises, to be on a par with female social class, but the numbers of men go down. Overall the social class of Edinburgh pharmacists rises as a result of the changes. Female entry is associated with processes making male and female entrants more similar and pharmacists of higher class. The more we find out about the process of entry the less adequate "feminisation" seems as a description, or "de-skilling" as an explanation.

This is also apparent in national data. Increasing numbers of women are part of a pattern that sees the age structure of working pharmacists transformed. Table 2 shows the age structure of UK working pharmacists for four separate years. In 1963, 45% of employed pharmacists were aged 50 or over. In 1987, in almost a complete reversal over 50% were under the age of 40. Pharmacy has not just undergone change in gender composition it has also developed from an older male profession to a much younger, more female one.

TABLE 2: Age Distribution of Working UK Pharmacists

Percentage in Age Group: Selected Years

AGE GROUP	1963	1969	1978	1987
under 30	16	14	20	28
30–39	16	21	22	23
40–49	23	15	22	20
50–59	30	29	13	15
over 60	16	22	23	14
TOTAL	100 (20,581)	100 (23,712)	100 (23,314)	100 (26,297)

Calculated from tables in *The Pharmaceutical Journal* 1964: 124, 1969: 615, 1978: 424, 1987: 224.

It seems that female entry is bound up with change in the status of the profession, and this has a knock-on effect on the class of the entrants. Change is not just from male to female pharmacists, but also to younger, more highly qualified, higher class incumbents who work in an occupation whose labour market and professional status has substantially altered. Pharmacy declines as an avenue for working class males who are squeezed out by changing educational requirements. The class origins of women stay the same with that of men becoming more similar. Employment re-structuring increases part-time and employee positions at the expense of ownership. So exactly at the point at which there is a demand for professional incumbents the ability of the occupational structure to support professional career development over the life course is weakened.

Clearly, the process of change over time is connected with changes in age and class structure in the profession as well as gender. Changes in gender composition are indivisible from these other changes. It is also apparent that at any one point in time, gender differences in employment encompass variation within gender categories that need to be incorporated into explanations. The concentration on gender divisions has generated too narrow a theoretical focus and emphasised particular divisions at the expense of others. Whilst it is vital to explain why women tend to be in lower status and lower paid jobs, this is not the same as arguing that pharmacy exhibits sex segregation. It is not clear that "gender segregation" is an accurate description of such patterns.

Crompton and Sanderson[3] see a gendered division of labour in pharmacy because women are generally in worse positions than men, and because they see characteristically "female" working patterns in female pharmacists' flexible part-time working. This can be seen by looking at the employment distributions of the Edinburgh sample in Table 3. This permits more detailed employment breakdowns than are possible from looking at national statistics. The Table breaks down distributions by part-time and full-time working, and only shows

TABLE 3: Employment Distribution by Sex and Hours of Working
(Edinburgh Sample)

Employment position	Males FT	Males PT	Females FT	Females PT	TOTAL	% OF MEN	% OF WOMEN
Hospital Employee	8 (35)		13 (57)	2 (9)	23 (101)	14	20
Chain Employee	7 (35)	1 (5)	4 (20)	8 (40)	20 (100)	14	16
Independent Employee	3 (10)	6 (19)	2 (7)	20 (65)	31 (101)	15	29
Owner	25 (54)	2 (4)	14 (30)	5 (11)	46 (99)	46	25
Industry	7 (70)		1 (10)	2 (20)	10 (100)	12	4
University			3 (67)	1 (33)	4 (100)		5
TOTAL	50 (37)	9 (7)	37 (28)	38 (28)	134 (100)	100	100

Figures in brackets represent row percentages. Also shows percentages in different employment positions broken down by sex. (FT = full-time, PT = part-time)

the pattern for the over 30s, in an attempt to compare like with like. Clearly, there is a skewed distribution by sex. Nearly half of the men are owners whilst only a quarter of women are. Given that women represent 57% of the over 30s they are very much under-represented in ownership. Similarly, over half the women are in part-time work, but few men are. However, Table 3 shows other important variation which needs to be incorporated into analysis.

Writers on the professions have indicated that important career development occurs in the early 30s and this is often the stage at which women miss out. Table 3 looks at older women, who are more established in their careers and are more likely to have made key transitions. These women are split between full-time work in hospitals, part-time work in the community sector and ownership. How are we to explain these important differences in the experience of women? Or that 40% of the owners – the best paid position and the destination of most older men – are female? Not in terms of gender divisions. The Table is the outcome of key movements made by both women and men as they age. The direction of this movement is away from the career structures of the hospital service and retail chains and into part-time work or ownership. Whilst there is a gender skew in these movements there is also a significant similarity in achievement of the most prestigious and advantaged forms of employment. Women do move into part-time work, more so than men, but, like men, a substantial number move into ownership. If differences are characterised as 'gender divisions' important variation within and across gender remains unexamined. The processes which generate differences also determine which women escape the relatively disadvantaged position of "women" in the profession, and which men have not realised the relative advantage of "men" in pharmacy.

CONCLUSION

The entry of women into pharmacy coincides with changes in the nature of employment relationships in general within the profession and can only be understood in this wider context. In particular, the relationship between the range of employment opportunities and the class, education and age of pharmacists undergoes a transformation which corresponds with, but cannot be reduced to, developments in gender composition. Because of the inter-related nature of these changes the meaning of the occupational title itself undergoes transformation. Pharmacists were once predominantly lower middle-class, apprentice-served men owning or working in small pharmacies. Now they have a higher social background, higher qualifications, are younger, more likely to be female and work in a much greater range of employment relationships.

The argument of this chapter is that a concentration on gender divisions in male-dominated professions has generated theoretical accounts of women's position which are misleading and unable to deal with the complexity of relationships. To see gender subordination or segregation as the main process of female entry to pharmacy is to mis-understand this process. Female entry, whilst skewed and associated with the re-structuring of opportunities, also occurs in a situation of employment advantage where a substantial number of women are achieving the most privileged positions. The *feminisation* of pharmacy is one strand in a transformation of relationships within the profession. Pharmacists and pharmacy have a much more diverse identity.

ACKNOWLEDGEMENT

This chapter is a modified version of a paper which was first published in *Work, Employment and Society* 1992; 6:329-349.

REFERENCES

1. Carter M, Carter S. Women's recent progress in professions or, women get a ticket after the gravy train has left the station. *Feminist Studies* 1981; 7: 477-504.
2. Crompton R, Sanderson K. Credentials and careers: some implications of the increase in professional qualifications amongst women. *Sociology* 1986; 20: 25-42.
3. Crompton R, Sanderson K. *Gendered Jobs and Social Change*. London: Unwin Hyman; 1990.
4. Kaufman D. Professional women: how real are the recent gains? In: Freeman J. ed. *Women: a feminist perspective*. Palo Alto: Mayfield; 1984.
5. Sokoloff N. The increase in black and white women in the professions: a contradictory process. In: Bose C, Spitze G. eds. *Ingredients for women's employment policy*. Albany: SUNY; 1987.
6. Reskin B, Roos P. Status hierarchies and sex segregation. In: Bose C, Spose G. eds. Op cit 1987.
7. Prandy K. The Revised Cambridge scale and sex segregation. *Sociology* 1990; 24: 629-655.

CHAPTER FOUR

RECORD KEEPING AND THE PROFESSIONALISATION OF COMMUNITY PHARMACY

Nicky Britten

INTRODUCTION

Computerised patient medication records (PMRs) have been used in community pharmacy in the UK since the mid 1980s; manual systems have been used for much longer. Stevens has described how computers were introduced to produce printed drug labels, and how the software to run PMR systems was developed later.[1] This eased the workload problems which had constrained manual systems of record keeping. The 1986 Nuffield report on pharmacy emphasised the importance of good record keeping and argued that services for patients on long term or complicated medication should be paid for separately.[2] The White Paper "Promoting Better Health"[3] published the same year endorsed this recommendation and advocated the keeping of patient medication records. Two years later the Department of Health announced that it would provide training courses in the introduction and maintenance of PMRs and would make payments to pharmacists who kept such records. It was estimated that 62% of community pharmacies were maintaining PMR systems in 1991 and that this figure might rise as high as 85% in the near future.[4]

Although one writer identified as many as 21 advantages offered by a PMR system,[5] the five main functions are as follows: detection of prescription errors; prevention of drug interactions; detection of adverse drug reactions; prevention of contraindicated medication due to allergies or disease; detection and prevention of misuse of drugs, both overuse and underuse. Some of these functions require a continuous record of previous prescriptions and some require information about the customer's clinical history. The PMR system is usually an integral part of the pharmacy's computer system, which also controls its stock and the labelling of medicines.

These functions combine to form a system of drug surveillance. This was a term defined in 1977 by the Dutch Working Group on Medication Surveillance:[6]

"Medication surveillance – conducted both by the physician and the pharmacist (in principle, each working separately on the basis of his tasks and responsibilities) – is the collection and organisation of information concerning the patient, including that of previously supplied medications, in order to judge whether the use of a particular drug: (1) carries the least possible risk for the patient, and (2) can result in optimal pharmacotherapy".

The above definition describes the function of PMR systems with the exception that doctors neither organise nor contribute to them. Doctors may use PMR systems as a resource to help them in their decision-making but, with the exception of a few pilot schemes, they do not contribute information to them except indirectly via the prescription.

To fulfil these surveillance functions, a PMR system must record certain items of information. The Department of Health payment scheme requires pharmacists to record the patient's name and address, the name, quantity and doses of drugs supplied on prescription and the date of supply.[7] However the Royal Pharmaceutical Society recommends recording of the following additional data: the patient's National Health Service number; sex; date of birth; telephone number; the name of the general practitioner; drug sensitivities and allergies; and chronic conditions.[8] The discrepancy between the Department's requirements and the Society's guidelines suggest that the latter is more concerned with the quality of the professional service provided.

THE PROFESSIONAL STATUS OF PHARMACY

The use of PMRs may be conceptualised as one aspect of the status of pharmacy as a profession. To explore this idea further it is first necessary to discuss the sociological analysis of the professions.

In common parlance the term 'profession' refers to certain occupations such as medicine or law, and not to certain other occupations such as shopkeeping or hairdressing. Sociologists have long wanted to know what distinguishes professional from non- professional occupations, and how certain occupational groups come to be defined as professions. Early sociological literature described how professions functioned to maintain the status quo and ensure the smooth running of society.[9] This approach led to the identification of a number of attributes (or traits) which seemed characteristic of professional occupations – such as specialist knowledge, an ethic of service to the community, extensive training, and licensing.[10] However, this type of explanation does not explain how certain groups came to be defined as professions or protected their professional status against the claims of other occupational groups. Wright's analysis of the rivalry between medicine and astrology in seventeenth century England showed that the failure of astrology was not a result of its inadequate knowledge base, but rather that it reflected the political power of medicine, and the compatibility of medical ideas with dominant ideas of the period.[11]

The importance of political power was reflected in Freidson's now classic analysis of the medical profession. It was the claim to clinical autonomy, he maintained, that protected doctors from outside interference, and was in its turn justified by three claims. First, it was argued that their skill and knowledge were so esoteric that outsiders were not equipped to evaluate it. Second, it was argued that professionals were responsible enough to work conscientiously without supervision. The third justification was that the profession had proper regulatory procedures to identify and control those of its members who fell below accepted standards. Freidson also examined relationships between occupational groups, and described how the medical profession came to exert control over the division of labour, to the detriment of paramedical occupations.[12] Nevertheless, there are grounds for believing that this medical control has declined in recent years as other health workers have pursued a professionalising strategy.[13]

Sociologists writing about pharmacy have sought to determine whether or not pharmacy is a profession. Denzin and Mettlin[14] argued that pharmacy was an example of incomplete professionalisation. By this they meant that although pharmacy possessed many of the attributes of a profession, it occupied a marginal position because it also contained elements of an occupation. These occupational, non-professional, elements included advertising, lack of altruism, a lack of monopoly on knowledge and, most importantly in the present context, failure to exert control over the social object they worked with, namely the drug. To describe the drug as a social object is to shift attention from its pharmacological nature. The social relationships between pharmacists, doctors and patients are partly determined by their different roles in relation to drugs, and drugs can thus be construed as social objects as well as pharmacological ones. The failure to exert control over drugs was, at least in part, based on the dominance of doctors in managing drug regimens. In respect of prescription drugs, a pharmacist may merely question the prescription if he or she believes it to be mistaken, and in some countries is allowed to substitute generic drugs for brand name prescriptions. The pharmacist has greater control over Pharmacy and General Sales List Medicines but these by definition are less potent. Moreover, although doctors have near exclusive control over prescribing (the advent of nurse prescribing not withstanding), pharmacists do not have exclusive control over dispensing, as some doctors in rural areas also have dispensing rights.

Denzin and Mettlin[14] also stressed the potential conflict between the drug as an object to be sold and as an object to which a service is directed. The profit motive encourages the sale of as many drugs as possible whereas a service orientation might result in lower consumption. In their discussion of incomplete professionalisation, Denzin and Mettlin characterise retail pharmacists as representing the most non-professional aspects of the profession.[14] A further factor undermining the professional status of pharmacists is increased automation.[15] Large scale manufacturing has replaced the compounding of drugs by individual pharmacists, and more and more drugs are dispensed in manufacturers' original packs. More generally, it is the conflict between community pharmacists' professional function and their commercial interests which weakens their claim to professional status. Part of the problem is that the public, and indeed doctors, may not perceive the pharmacist as having a specialist knowledge of drugs or as offering a professional service, despite pharmacists' self perceptions to the contrary.

Discussion of the impediments to pharmacy achieving full professional status can easily be seen as a rather static analysis. But the situation may be seen as much more dynamic, especially viewed in its historical context. Power struggles in nineteenth century England between physicians, surgeons, apothecaries, chemists and druggists eventually resulted in the present division between medicine and pharmacy. Today's descendant of the apothecary is not the pharmacist but the general practitioner, who still retains the right to dispense in certain circumstances. The chemists and druggists took over the tasks of compounding and dispensing medicines, largely abandoned by the apothecaries, and their descendants are today's pharmacists. They were left with fairly technical tasks, which have in turn been threatened by the automation of much of present day pharmacy. To counter this threat to their status pharmacists have begun to redefine the role of pharmacy.

The development of the pharmaceutical industry in the twentieth century has resulted in large numbers of new drugs, (many of which are virtually indistinguishable from one another), combination-drug products, in serious adverse effects, not to mention the aggressive marketing and promotion of new drugs.[16] These changes increase the possibility of prescription errors, drug interactions and adverse effects. In response, it has been possible to define a new clinical role for pharmacy, which consists of detecting these same prescribing errors, monitoring drug interactions and adverse effects, and providing advice and guidance on drugs to both patients and doctors. The new role has been described as clinical pharmacy in relation to hospital practice and as an extended role in relation to community pharmacy. In both cases the new role represents the definition of a new area of clinical activity for pharmacists. Eaton and Webb[17] referred to this redefinition as 'boundary encroachment', maintaining that clinical pharmacy is an attempt to extend the boundaries of pharmacy practice into the territory of the medical profession, the boundary in this case being that between prescribing and dispensing. Eaton and Webb maintained that the success or failure of the clinical pharmacy movement depended on the reaction of the medical profession and concluded that a negotiated settlement had been reached. Pharmacists have accepted the fact that doctors have ultimate responsibility for the patient but in exchange for this acceptance they have acquired the right to practice certain activities on the periphery of clinical medicine. Pharmacists usually refrain from doing anything that would damage the doctor's reputation in the eyes of the patient. There is an agreement not to threaten or trespass upon significant medical activities. As a result of this, expansion of the boundaries of pharmacy into clinical areas has not corresponded with any decline in medical dominance of paramedical occupations. Such restriction of doctors' autonomy as has occurred has been brought about by the Government, for example when introducing the Limited List of prescribable drugs, and not by pharmacists. Eaton and Webb argued that the new roles adopted by pharmacy such as patient counselling and the provision of drug information services are those neglected by doctors. Indeed in an analysis of clinical pharmacy in two American hospitals, Mesler noted that some doctors were glad to relinquish the burden of keeping up to date with drug technology.[18]

To summarise, in sociological terms, although clinical pharmacy and the extended role are part of an attempt to increase the professional standing of pharmacy, the continued subservience of pharmacy to the medical profession prevents it achieving full professional status.

PATIENT MEDICATION RECORDS AND THE PHARMACIST'S EXTENDED ROLE

Harding, Nettleton and Taylor[19] identified twelve components of the pharmacist's extended role ranging from advising patients on minor ailments to diagnostic testing. Record keeping is an essential part of the new role and one on which several of the other components depend, such as providing advice on the use of medicines and the monitoring of adverse reactions.

If the pharmacist's extended role involves boundary encroachment, then record keeping might be said to be situated on the boundary. The detection of prescription errors requires either that the prescription be returned to the doctor for rewriting or that the pharmacist corrects the error after contacting the prescriber. Either way the pharmacist is influencing the act of prescribing. The detection of interactions may suggest that one of the drugs in question be altered: again this influences prescribing. The detection of adverse drug reactions or contraindications might result in the patient seeking a further consultation with the doctor, with some specific advice from the pharmacist about future drug choices. The detection of misuse of drugs might also affect prescribing: in the case of overuse, by reducing the level of prescribing and in the case of underuse, by suggesting the need for a different drug or a different therapeutic approach.

Record keeping as a boundary activity is more than an influence on prescribing; it also performs a surveillance function as community pharmacists are in a position to monitor general practitioners' prescribing habits whether they keep records or not. For example, the recent case of a general practitioner who prescribed bizarre items such as hair shampoo for internal consumption and creosote was brought to public notice by the local pharmacist.[20] Record keeping however extends these possibilities by enabling the pharmacist to detect inadvertent changes of dose or interactions between drugs prescribed at different times, for example. This is a different type of surveillance from the one quoted earlier in this chapter, which referred to surveillance of the patient by doctor and pharmacist. Surveillance of prescribing habits is to a small extent a curb on the doctor's clinical autonomy and constitutes regulation from outside the medical profession. The fact that both doctor and pharmacist are responsible for ensuring that the patient receives appropriate medication is confirmed by legal rulings in which the exact proportion of responsibility attributed to each party is calculated.[19] Unlike other forms of record keeping, PMRs are not a good method of scrutinising the work of the record keeper, but the keeping of PMRs is thus a method of surveillance of both doctor and patient. In a sociological account of record keeping, Rees discussed the construction of hospital records.[21] He pointed out that the record says as much about the person who wrote it as about the patient. Thus, the junior hospital doctors who do most of the clerking of new patients are aware that their seniors may judge them on the quality of their record keeping.[21] In a different setting, Freidson pointed out that doctors' records are visible in a way that their clinical performance is not, but suggested that the medical record becomes a supervisory device only if interest has been generated, for example by a complaint, otherwise medical records are not scrutinised routinely.[22] The reasons that PMRs are not useful devices for scrutinising the work of pharmacists is that they are optional, that they are kept in a machine defined format which allows for less creativity on the part of the pharmacist, and that patients' use of several pharmacies may render records incomplete. In respect of the latter point, it is possible that just as the keeping of PMRs can affect doctors' prescribing behaviour, it may also affect patient behaviour. If patients are aware that a particular pharmacy keeps computerised records and are averse to computer databases, they may deliberately avoid going to that pharmacy. If they perceive the PMR as improving the personal service offered by a pharmacy, this may increase their loyalty. Jepson et al, in a survey of customers' expectations of community pharmacy, found that personal service was a major factor in customer loyalty.[23]

Two further aspects of record keeping discussed by Rees are relevant here.[21] First, he pointed out that the opening of a record creates a link between the individual and an organisation, so that the creation of a hospital record is part of the process of becoming a patient. In the same way, the opening of a computerised record creates a link between a customer and a particular pharmacy. This link may be reinforced by the issuing of a medication record card held by the customer, to be presented to the pharmacist whenever a prescription is to be dispensed. Second, Rees pointed out that record keeping is seen as an irksome and boring activity. The workload involved in setting up and keeping PMR systems has been much discussed in *The Pharmaceutical Journal* especially in relation to payment. Many pharmacists do not feel that the amount paid by the Department of Health is adequate for the amount of work involved. This is of course part of the wider question of payment for the pharmacist's professional services. Most of the activities which make up the extended role are not ones for which pharmacists are paid, and may take time away from their income generating activities.

The tension between community pharmacists' commercial interests and professionalism was referred to earlier. The PMR is part of both the professional and the commercial functions of community pharmacy. The same computer system can be used to generate labels for customers, control stock, store a pharmaceutical database, and keep PMRs. Holloway *et al.*[24] suggest that the professional and commercial functions of pharmacy do not necessarily conflict. It may be that the maintenance of high professional standards is a good commercial strategy which enhances patient loyalty in the long term. The idea of patient registration, which would lead to more complete and therefore better patient records, is opposed by those pharmacists who fear that the protection from competition thus afforded might lead to a lowering of professional standards. It is instructive to consider the situation elsewhere. In the Netherlands, pharmacists do not have to sell non pharmaceutical products. Because of Sick Fund requirements, the majority of the population were until recently required to register with a pharmacy and customer loyalty is still strong. Pharmacists undergo a longer training than in the UK and are held in greater esteem by doctors. The exchange of information between doctor and pharmacist is accepted practice, and the pharmacist is accepted as an unbiased adviser on drug issues. About 90% of pharmacists keep computerised record systems and make them available to doctors.[6] In this situation therefore good practice in record keeping has gone hand in hand with professionalism in pharmacy and high social esteem. Despite claims to the contrary, the Netherlands experience suggests that professionalism in pharmacy is enhanced by a non commercial environment.

THE USER'S PERSPECTIVE

The relatively harmonious situation in the Netherlands obscures problems which may be more troublesome elsewhere. One of the main obstacles to good practice in record keeping in the UK is the incompleteness of the records arising from the patients' right to use more than one pharmacy for the dispensing of prescriptions. The introduction of smart cards was intended to address this problem, but patients do not always remember to carry them,[25] and their future is uncertain. There has been little attempt to research patients' understanding or expectations of PMR or smart card systems. This lack of interest in the patients' view is shown not only in regard to smart card use but also in the sociological discussion of the professions. It is only as the concept of consumerism in medicine has developed that patients' preferences have become the subject of research interest.[26] Some writers have argued that increased consumerism will result in the deprofessionalisation of medicine, and as pharmacy already operates in a consumer market, it is more susceptible than medicine to the opinion of its customers.

Jepson *et al* found that customers, especially those identified as high users of pharmacy services, liked the idea of PMR systems.[23] They also found that customers were often unaware that the pharmacy they used kept PMRs. These findings were similar to those of Britten *et al*[27] who found that customers were in favour of PMRs but not necessarily aware of their potential advantages. Such awareness as existed was associated with the holding of a medication record card or personal experience of the PMR system. In this study some patients were reluctant to give pharmacists their medical histories because they considered it unnecessary, since either the pharmacist could infer it from the medication or the doctor already had the details. Respondents appeared to think that there was considerable exchange of information between doctors and pharmacists, and that doctors' records were bound to be complete and correct. These results suggest that pharmacists need to inform their customers of the PMR system, both by issuing medication record cards and by making it clear that the record has been consulted before dispensing a prescription. Ideally customers should be aware of the potential benefits of PMR systems, but as several of these benefits carry the implication that doctors sometimes make mistakes, this may be difficult for individual pharmacists. When asking for details of a customer's medical history, pharmacists need to make it clear why such information is necessary and why it is presently unavailable from other sources.

The role of the medical profession in restricting or encouraging the pharmacist's clinical role has been much discussed by sociologists and others. However the extended role also requires the customer's cooperation and acceptance. The potential for the failure of PMR and other systems of record keeping may not come from hostile doctors but from customers unaware of the potential benefits of the pharmacist's extended role for themselves.

REFERENCES

1. Stevens R. The evolution of patient medication records in British community pharmacy. *International Journal of Pharmacy Practice* 1991; 1: 64-72.
2. Nuffield Committee of Inquiry into Pharmacy. *Pharmacy: A report to the Nuffield Foundation*. London: The Nuffield Foundation; 1986.
3. *Promoting Better Health Care: an agenda for discussion*. Cmd 9771 London: HMSO; 1986.
4. Rogers PJ, Fletcher G, Rees JE. Patient medication records in community pharmacy. *The Pharmaceutical Journal* 1992; 248: 193-196.
5. Morris G. Patient medication records: a personal view. *The Pharmaceutical Journal* 1989; 242: 351-2.
6. Van Gruting CWD, de Gier JJ. Medication assistance: the development of drug surveillance and drug information in the Netherlands. *The Annals of Pharmacotherapy* 1992; 26: 1008-1012.
7. *Drug Tariff: National Health Service, England and Wales*. London: HMSO; 1991.
8. *The Pharmaceutical Journal* 1989; 242: 348.
9. Parsons T. *The Social System*. London: Free Press; 1951.
10. Goode WJ. Encroachment, charlatanism and the emerging profession: psychiatry, sociology and medicine. *American Sociological Review* 1960; 25: 902-914.
11. Wright PWG. A study in the legitimisation of knowledge: the 'success' of medicine and the 'failure' of astrology. In: Wallis R. ed. *On the margins of science: the social construction of rejected knowledge*. Sociological Review Monograph 27: University of Keele; 1979.
12. Freidson E. *Profession of medicine: a study in the sociology of applied knowledge*. New York: Dodd, Mead and Company; 1975.
13. Armstrong D. The decline of the medical hegemony: a review of government reports during the NHS. *Social Science and Medicine* 1976; 10: 157-163.
14. Denzin NK, Mettlin CJ. Incomplete professionalization: the case of pharmacy. *Social Forces* 1968; 46: 375-381.
15. Birenbaum A. Reprofessionalization in pharmacy. *Social Science and Medicine* 1982; 16: 871-878.
16. Mechanic D. Social issues in the study of the pharmaceutical field. *American Journal of Pharmaceutical Education* 1970; 34: 536-543.
17. Eaton G, Webb B. Boundary encroachment: pharmacists in the clinical setting. *Sociology of Health and Illness* 1979; 1: 69-89.
18. Mesler MA. Boundary encroachment and task delegation: clinical pharmacists on the medical team. *Sociology of Health and Illness* 1991; 13: 310-331.
19. Harding G, Nettleton S, Taylor K. *Sociology for pharmacists: an introduction*. Basingstoke: Macmillan; 1990.
20. *The Guardian* 7 October 1992.
21. Rees C. Records and hospital routine. In: Atkinson P, Heath C. eds. *Medical work: realities and routines*. Farnborough: Gower; 1981.
22. Freidson E. *Medical Work in America: Essays on Health Care*. New Haven: Yale University Press; 1989.

23. Jepson M, Jesson J, Kendall H, Pocock R. *Consumer expectations of community pharmaceutical services: a research report for the Department of Health.* Birmingham: MEL Aston University; 1991.
24. Holloway SWF, Jewson ND, Mason DJ. 'Reprofessionalization' or 'occupational imperialism'?: some reflections on pharmacy in Britain. *Social Science and Medicine* 1986; 23: 323-332.
25. *The Pharmaceutical Journal* 1991; 246: 43.
26. Haug MR. The deprofessionalisation of everyone? *Sociological Focus* 1975; 3: 197-213.
27. Britten N, Gallagher K, Gallagher H. Patients' views of computerised pharmacy records. *International Journal of Pharmacy Practice* 1992; 1: 206-209.

CHAPTER FIVE

WORKING FOR HEALTH: INTERPROFESSIONAL RELATIONS IN HEALTH CENTRES

Geoffrey Harding, Kevin Taylor and Sarah Nettleton

INTRODUCTION

Successful provision of health services to the public requires communication, co-operation and collaboration between members of the primary health care team. However, a number of factors may inhibit effective co-operation between health professionals, such as differences in the status, prestige and power of the respective team members.[1] Additionally, inadequate communication and poor appreciation of each other's roles have been suggested as hindering the development of a more team-based approach to health care.[2] One strategy which aims to promote the concept of the community based health care team is the centralisation of health services into one location. Health centres provide a structure for such centralisation and potential co-operation (fig 1.). They provide a physical location for key health professionals such as general practitioners, practice nurses, midwives and health visitors, in addition to other health personnel such as chiropodists, dentists, opticians and pharmacists. Health centres also impose a structure within which professional responsibilities and thresholds are clearly defined, as distinct from the situation in the "community", where developments such as doctor dispensing, nurse prescribing and the concept of the pharmacist's extended role have led to a redefinition of roles and a blurring of the boundaries demarcating each health profession's domain.

Health centres as we know them were first defined in the Dawson Report of 1920,[3] as institutions "...wherein are brought various medical services, both preventative and curative, so as to form one organisation". Provision of a national network of health centres was envisaged in the original plans for the National Health Service in the United Kingdom. Indeed, the National Health Service Act of 1946 charged local authorities with responsibility for providing,

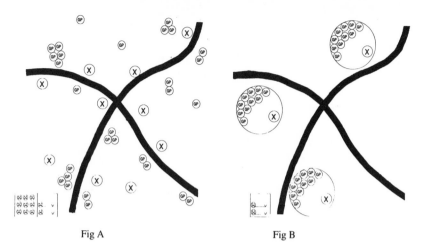

Fig A   Fig B

GP = General Practitioner, X = Other health care professionals, ⊗ = Hospital Out-Patients, ⟁⤳ =
Hospital In-Patients. In the traditional set up illustrated in fig A: general practitioners work singly
or in groups. The hospital (bottom left) has out-patient and in-patient deparments overflowing
with patients. In Fig B: the chaotic arrangements for health care are rationalised into health
centres, in which general practitioners and other health professionals work together. Much of the
work previously handled by the hospital is now based in the health centre. (Adapted from Draper
P, Community Care Units: What Should be Done. *Medical World* 1969; 107:4)

Figure 1: Diagramatic representation of rationale behind location of health
professionals

equipping and staffing health centres, bringing together health professionals to
provide health, and in particular, preventative services. However, by 1958 only
ten such centres had been constructed, due to difficulties in attracting the
participation of general practitioners who were already forming themselves into
group practices.[4]

In the late 1960s interest in health centres was rekindled, such that in 1968
there were 110 centres compared to 60 in the previous year.[5] This dramatic
increase resulted from difficulties in providing premises for group practices of
general practitioners, combined with the need to provide health services to the
populations of new housing estates.

The Nuffield Inquiry into Pharmacy[6] suggested that providing
pharmaceutical services in health centres should encourage the formation of
close links between pharmacists and other health care professionals. One of the
aims of the study reported here was to assess whether or not closer links were
established between these practitioners. However, at present few community
pharmacists work in health centres. In fact less than 2% of the approximately
10,000 community pharmacies in England are located in health centres, as
defined by the Department of Health.

Prior to the study reported here, it was not known whether including a pharmacy in the fabric of a health centre had a marked or even measurable impact on the relationship between pharmacists, general practitioners and other health workers. Clearly, the close physical proximity of health personnel enhances the potential for interprofessional collaboration and it may be postulated that a mutual exchange of expertise naturally follows. However, it is also possible that such exchange of expertise may be perceived as a dilution of a professional knowledge base and be subsequently resisted. Antagonism based on perceptions of status may also be exacerbated.

These and other issues were addressed in a study of all (101) health centre pharmacies in England, conducted in 1988.[7-11] The study sought to characterise health centre pharmacies and evaluate the impact close physical proximity had on pharmacists' relations with other health personnel, in particular general practitioners.

PROFESSIONALISATION AND INTERPROFESSIONAL RELATIONS

The nature of relations between occupational groups within the context of health care in general and in health care centres in particular has been subject to extensive sociological scrutiny and debate.[12,13] The limited effectiveness of teamwork given differences in status and power between professional groups has also been documented.[1,14,15] The "occupational control" thesis argues that within the health care division of labour the medical profession is dominant in relation to other professional groups, who are deemed to be "para-professionals."[16] The work of such para-professionals is limited by the dominant medical profession. For example, pharmacists dispense medication in accordance with the instructions of the prescribing doctors. Such features of the relations between professional groups are fundamental if we are to make sense of the quality of the interactions between pharmacists and doctors.

The nature of the work and the status of general practitioners and pharmacists have changed in recent years with both occupational groups attaining greater social status (see chapters 3 and 4). General practitioners for example, until the 1970s were a relatively marginalised group within the medical profession. However, more recently, they have reasserted their professional status largely through a recourse to "biographical medicine" that is, an approach to care which emphasises the patient as a "whole" person.[17] General practitioners are required to be well versed in communication and interpretative skills which designate them as "experts" in a particular type of medicine.

The activities of pharmacists have also changed. In terms of professional status however, it may be argued that they remain a para-professional group: their status as "professionals" being hindered by a number of factors such as, the commercial context of their work, the process of deskilling as a result of pre-formulated and pre-packaged drugs, the fragmentation of pharmacy into occupations ranging from retail managers, industrial chemists and administrators, and the subordination of the hospital pharmacist to the medical profession.[18] However, recent initiatives, such as the enhanced involvement of pharmacists in drug therapy on hospital wards (see chapter 14), "ask your pharmacist" campaigns promoting pharmacists as advisors on minor ailments, and the location of pharmacists within health centres have promoted their direct involvement with patients, and therefore their capacity to function as "health care" practitioners has increased. There is also a recognition within pharmacy education (see chapters 15 and 16) that prospective pharmacists require skills for patient orientated tasks and a biographical approach to care.

Whilst the content of pharmacists' work may be changing they have not challenged the medical profession's authority to define the agenda. Such differences in status between these two groups will influence their interactions and interpersonal relations. These issues have been explored within health centres.

To construct a profile of health centre pharmacies: their locality, physical features, personnel etc. and compare them to a broadly matched group of community pharmacists, a questionnaire survey was conducted. The questionnaires were sent to the managers (all pharmacists) of every English health centre pharmacy and to an equal number of community pharmacy managers. The latter group of pharmacies were comparable to the health centre pharmacies in terms of monthly prescription turnover and location within the same Family Health Services Authority (FHSA). Usable questionnaires were received from 93 (92%) and 90 (89%) of health centre and community pharmacy managers respectively.

FINDINGS

The inclusion of pharmacies within health centres was a recent development, with 70% opening since 1977. More than two thirds (68%) of health centre pharmacies opened at the same time as the health centre, and a further 16% opened within one year of the centre's opening. The distribution of health centre pharmacies throughout England showed marked geographical variation. There was a very large proportion of the total number in the north of the country, Lancashire alone had 31 such pharmacies, whilst there were very few in the South, with the whole of the South East having only 3. Sixty three per cent of the health centres with pharmacies were situated in urban areas, i.e. in a town or shopping precinct; 34% had a suburban situation, in mainly residential areas away from shopping areas. Only 3% were situated in a rural environment.

The dispensary area comprised at least half the available floor space in 94% of health centre pharmacies, whilst in 65% of cases the dispensary monopolised virtually all the floor space. This compared to 55% of community pharmacies in which the dispensary occupied less than half the available floor space. This clearly reflects the nature of the business conducted in each type of pharmacy, which is further indicated by the products available for purchase from the pharmacies. Over the counter medicines were available at all but 4% of health centre pharmacies. However, only 37% offered a wide selection of such medication, with 59% offering a limited selection. All community pharmacies supplied over the counter medicines with 97% offering a wide selection. Non-medical merchandise which was available from virtually all (97%) community pharmacies was only obtainable from 49% of health centre pharmacies.

There was an approximately balanced distribution of male (56%) and female (44%) managers in health centre pharmacies. In community pharmacies, however, there was a greater imbalance with the ratio of male to female managers greater than 2 to 1 (72% and 28% respectively). On the whole female health centre pharmacy managers were younger than their male counterparts. Fifty one per cent of female managers were aged less than 35 years compared to 42% for their male counterparts.

On average, excluding locums, there were 1.3 pharmacists and 2 dispensing technicians employed per health centre pharmacy compared to 1.5 pharmacists and 1.3 dispensing technicians per community pharmacy. This gives a pharmacist to technician ratio of 1:1.5 and 1:0.9 in health centre and community pharmacies respectively. However, community pharmacies had many more non-dispensing assistants (3.7 per pharmacy) than health centre pharmacies (0.7 per pharmacy).

Not surprisingly perhaps, such physical proximity to one another did yield a

TABLE 1: Frequency of pharmacist's consultations by general practitioners
(Adapted from reference 8)

	Frequency of Consultation	
	Health centre pharmacists (%)	Community pharmacists (%)
30 times per week or more	9.7	5.0
10–29 times per week	36.5	21.7
Less than 10 times per week	47.3	48.9
Hardly ever	6.5	24.4

more frequent rate of general practitioner instigated consultations between the prescribers and the health centre pharmacists when compared to community pharmacists (Table 1). Fewer than one in ten health centre pharmacists (9.7%) were consulted by general practitioners on a frequent basis i.e. 30 times per week or more; though appreciably fewer community pharmacists were similarly consulted (5%). The greater proportion of health centre pharmacists (53.8%) were consulted by general practitioners on an occasional basis i.e. less than ten times per week, though again a comparatively greater proportion of community pharmacists (73.2%) received only occasional consultations from general practitioners. Similar trends were observed when pharmacists were asked about the frequency of consultation by health professionals other than general practitioners (Table 2).

TABLE 2: Frequency of pharmacist's consultations by health professionals other than general practitioners

	Frequency of Consultation	
	Health centre pharmacists (%)	Community pharmacists (%)
10 times per week or more	46.7	25.7
Less than 10 times per week	51.1	71.4
Hardly ever	2.2	2.9

The proportion of health centre pharmacy managers consulted ten times per week or more by such professionals was almost twice that of pharmacists practising in the community. The health professionals reported to consult with pharmacists are shown in Figure 2. For each profession the percentage of pharmacists reporting a consultation was greatest for those working in health centres. The difference between the two groups of pharmacists was greatest for health visitors, midwives and chiropodists, which probably reflects the high incidence of these professionals working within health centres.

One rationale for employing pharmacists in health centres is to promote pharmacist–general practitioner liaison. The data discussed above indicates that inclusion of a pharmacy does seem to increase the incidence of consultation. However, interviews with the respective health professionals indicated that organisational and structural barriers existed even within an integrated health centre, which inhibited pharmacist–general practitioner communication.

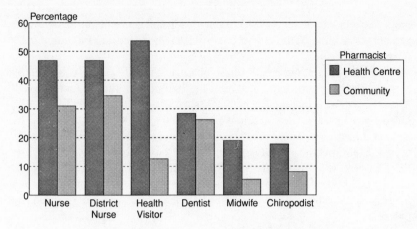

Figure 2: Health Professionals who consult with pharmacists.

One pharmacist commented:

> "Sometimes it's difficult to get through the receptionist to get to the doctor and I think it would be much more helpful if the doctor would recognise that we're trying to help them, trying to help the patients as well, and let us get at them (general practitioners) so we can talk to them personally. Basically I think (that it is) the receptionist who protects the doctor all the time."

Ironically, another observed that centralised health care organisations can actually have the opposite effect to that which is intended. For example, one pharmacist commented that he did not,

> "... see as much of them (general practitioners) as I'd like to. There's a tendency for group practices to have their own tea rooms, where as in the old days with single handed practices there was more opportunity to have informal chats."

Thus the practice was so organised that the doctors tended to keep themselves separate from the rest of the staff.

INTERPROFESSIONAL RELATIONS BETWEEN GENERAL PRACTITIONERS AND PHARMACISTS

In addition to collecting data on the physical properties of health centre pharmacies and the personnel employed within it, the questionnaire survey sought to establish in a basic way how the various health professionals, working in a shared environment, interacted with each other. To explore more deeply some aspects of the mechanics of the relationships and indeed their dynamics, interviews, using semi-structured interview schedules, were carried out with a sample drawn from those who participated in the questionnaire survey. Ten health centres having an integral pharmacy were selected for this part of the study, one from each of the Regional Health Authorities in England which possessed one or more such health centres. The pharmacy manager of each health centre was interviewed along with thirteen general practitioners – at least one from each health centre. For comparative purposes interviews, using suitably modified schedules, were conducted with ten community pharmacists and nine general practitioners working in health centres without pharmacies, located within the vicinity of the above health centres.

While the location of a pharmacy in a health centre may facilitate the development of interprofessional relations, whether or not this infrastructure is capitalised upon by personnel depends on further considerations. For example, respective perceptions of the other's professional role may determine whether professional co-operation and development is considered appropriate or indeed desirable. Interviews with general practitioners and pharmacists, both within health centres with and without integral pharmacies explored these considerations.

It was apparent that general practitioners readily utilised the pharmacist's close proximity, as one said for example:

> "...I go down and ask regularly when I've got a query. If I ever have a problem about drugs I always go down and ask them...I ring him far more often than he rings me...."

and another commented:

> "I often have queries about problems of prescribing details and I wouldn't hesitate to ring up any time to seek advice of the pharmacist..."

Six of the thirteen general practitioners interviewed indeed considered as routine, their face-to-face contact with the pharmacist. The remainder approached the pharmacists by telephone or through an intermediary such as a pharmacy assistant.

The pharmacists interviewed however, highlighted the fact they had to negotiate access to general practitioners through the reception staff and observed that this was as a significant factor which influenced the regularity of their contacts. The majority (8) reported that this was the usual route of contact with the general practitioner. Three pharmacists had direct telephone links with the general practitioner. Whilst only two reported that communication with general practitioners was either "face to face" or via telephone. Pharmacist-instigated "face to face" communication was reported to be difficult since their absence from the pharmacy had to be "covered".

In the main, general practitioners sought to consult health centre pharmacists on drug dosage and/or quantity: "I often have queries about problems of prescribing details and I wouldn't hesitate to ring up anytime to seek advice of the pharmacist." They also appreciated the pharmacists's input in ensuring the accuracy and appropriateness of their prescribing, as one general practitioner noted:

> "I find them very useful, I find it very comforting to have someone behind me making sure that I don't do something silly."

and,

> "Its a check on whether you're doing right or wrong",

and again,

> "Pleased that checking process is there."

Eleven of the thirteen general practitioners interviewed also believed health centre pharmacists influenced prescribing patterns by, for example recommending equally effective but cheaper generic rather than proprietary products. Community pharmacists were reported to influence the prescribing patterns of only 3 out of 9 general practitioners in health centres without pharmacies. Notwithstanding such recommendations, eight of the ten health centre pharmacists reported that their medical stock was determined by what the general practitioner prescribed, yet only four general practitioners appreciated they influenced the pharmacy's stock, while nine believed they did not. Thus the perceptions or definitions of any given situation can vary according to an individual's position within an organisational structure. An appreciation of professionals' own perceptions, articulated in their own words, is crucial to understanding any interprofessional relationships.

A particularly strong theme to emerge from the interviews with general practitioners and pharmacists was the often contradictory perceptions each had of their professional relationship. Although, with few exceptions, reports from both pharmacists and general practitioners tended to sum up their relationship as essentially satisfactory, further analysis revealed that the term "satisfactory" was in fact evoked in several ways to define the relationship. Descriptions of a "satisfactory" relationship indicate only a positive evaluation of relations, and was used in the limited sense, simply indicating that they happened to "get on" with one another: they had reasonable interpersonal relations and a working relationship which functioned relatively smoothly. Indeed some health centre pharmacists defined their relationship exclusively in these terms and made comments such as: "there's no reason why, it's just that we get on quite well" and "We're on friendly terms" and again "its a matter of relationships really. It's a good rapport between people". When these pharmacists described their relationship as satisfactory therefore, they were not referring to what might be considered the "professional" aspects of their relationship.

Some general practitioners in health centres with pharmacists defined their "satisfactory relationship' as one in which they could turn to the pharmacist in his or her capacity as an expert for advice. In such cases the pharmacist's specialist knowledge was made available on an equitable basis. As one general practitioner commented:

"I often have queries about problems of prescribing details and I wouldn't hesitate to ring up any time to seek advice of the pharmacist...and he's most helpful in that respect."

The general practitioners regarded the pharmacist's screening and checking role as the most important aspect of their relationship. In this respect given the pharmacist's responsibility to ensure that patients receive the appropriate prescribed medication, prescribers clearly considered the pharmacist's close working proximity could be advantageous. As one general practitioner observed:

"I would rely on her utterly to see that everything was all right because people (pharmacists) outside (of the health centre) would not know my habits as well..."

and another:

"I would expect this one (on site pharmacist) to know my pattern of prescribing...to know what to expect of me if there were some glaring error or mistake."

This "checking service" was valued by general practitioners over and above other potential contributions such as technical information and knowledge of drug costs. General practitioners expectations of "in house" pharmacists, although evaluated positively, were therefore generally limited to this one element. Pharmacists in health centres were more ambivalent about their professional relations with their general practitioner colleagues in health centres. For example, dissatisfaction was expressed when the potential for "professional" dialogue was not realised: as one health centre pharmacist put it:

"I feel it (the relationship) could be better, not from the point of view that we don't get on, but from the point of view that I think there should be more of a *professional relationship*...I would like to be more useful to them in cost effective prescribing...." [our emphasis]

This would suggest that the general practitioner either does not recognise or fails to exploit the pharmacist's wider specialist knowledge and skills. There is a sense of frustration that the general practitioner does not utilise the pharmacist's professional skills to compliment their own.

Perhaps the most constraining aspect to the relationship between pharmacists and general practitioners working in close proximity arose from concerns about possible boundary encroachment of one profession's domain by another. This was especially apparent among some general practitioners who expressed the view that pharmacists should not give anything but the simplest of advice to patients about their medication. For example, one doctor said,

"The pharmacist should give a brief broad based description of what drugs are doing, but shouldn't go into any detail"

and another elaborated further that he was;

"...uneasy about the idea of pharmacists dispensing medical knowledge for two reasons – lack of knowledge and patient history. By no stretch of the imagination could the pharmacist be considered to be competent medically....in practice a lot of the advice patients seem to get from pharmacists is not good advice....a pharmacist might be a very good pharmacist but I would feel uncomfortable about (him/her) giving advice on a cough."

CONCLUSION

Recent National Health Service (NHS) reforms redefine the traditional boundaries of professional responsibilities, in pursuit of cost efficient health services to patients. These reforms have clearly impacted upon pharmacy with, for instance, proposals for nurse prescribing and budget holding general practitioners. These reforms were instigated subsequent to the completion of this research. Consequently the views of general practitioners and pharmacists that we have reported, do not reflect this new structure. Nonetheless, it was evident from this research that although close working proximity encouraged exchanges between the two types of practitioner the content of such interactions were invariably limited to relatively unproblematic and non challenging issues such as cost effective prescribing, screening prescriptions prior to dispensing, or tailoring the pharmacy stock in accordance with prescribers' practices: issues, related to products rather than therapies, which do not as such impinge upon the professional boundaries of either pharmacists or general practitioners. The under-utilisation of pharmacists as "experts" in drug therapy has previously been reported by researchers in Australia and the United States of America.[19,20,21] These studies indicated that physicians were much more ready to accept product-related information from pharmacists than therapeutic information.

These exchanges were regarded by the medical practitioners as being the appropriate and indeed useful function of the pharmacists. Some of the pharmacists however felt that their function could be extended further and could be used more effectively. It is pertinent that none of the exchanges or interactions were such that they encroached on the doctors' professional boundary. More recent developments such as the introduction of patient medication records (see chapter 4) might well alter the nature of interprofessional interactions in this respect. In general it does appear that health centre based pharmacies have benefits which arise from increased proximity of pharmacists and general practitioners, and that pharmacists within such pharmacies are more likely to influence the prescribing patterns of general practitioners. In this context it is interesting to note that other research has suggested that prescribing costs are reduced as a result of more rational prescribing and prescribing in smaller quantities when general practitioners collaborate with pharmacists[22].

However proximity alone is only one contributory factor promoting interprofessional relations. Working under the same roof may forge satisfactory, if somewhat brittle, personal relations, but extending and developing interprofessional roles involves mutual recognition of the other's skills and expertise – particularly recognition by general practitioners of the pharmacist's skills and knowledge. Differential social status of general practitioners and pharmacists notwithstanding, the restructuring of the health service, with an increasing emphasis upon medical audit, cost effectiveness and quality assurance, provides pharmacists in health centres (as well as those in the community) with an opportunity to consolidate their role as the prescriber's drug "expert". Health centre pharmacists can influence general practitioners, for instance in assisting cost-effective prescribing. However, in order to develop their relationship with general practitioners in health centres, pharmacists should be more involved with patient care and not just promote themselves as an information source for cost-effective prescribing.

Health centres represent a microcosm of the reorganised community health services and have long been regarded as key sites for disease prevention and health promotion. The health centre serves to promote, as well as to restore, health and provides the infrastructure for general practitioners and pharmacists to work collaboratively within a framework of the new public health movement. A key to further collaboration in the future may therefore involve their mutual participation (with others) in establishing outcome measures with which to evaluate health centre based health promotion strategies.

ACKNOWLEDGEMENT

The research upon which this chapter is based was supported by a grant from the Department of Health.

REFERENCES

1. Bond J, Cartlidge AM, Gregson BA *et al*. Interprofessional collaboration in primary

health care. *Journal of the Royal College of General Practitioners* 1987; 37: 158-161.

2. Department of Health and Social Security. *Neighbourhood nursing: a focus for care* (Cumberlege Report). London: HMSO; 1986.

3. Ministry of Health Consultative Council and Allied Services. *Interim report on the future provision of medical and allied services.* London: HMSO (Cmd 693); 1920.

4. Ashworth HW. The failure of health centres. *Journal of the Royal College of General Practitioners* 1959; 8: 357-364.

5. Brookes B. The Historical Perspective in Health Centres, in Wise ARJ. ed. *British Health Care and Technology.* London: Health and Social Service Journal/Hospital International; 1974.

6. Nuffield Committee of Inquiry into Pharmacy. *Pharmacy: A report to the Nuffield Foundation.* London: Nuffield Foundation; 1986.

7. Harding G, Taylor KMG. Pharmacies in health centres. *Journal of the Royal College of General Practitioners* 1988; 38: 566-567.

8. Harding G, Taylor KMG. Health centre pharmacies in England. *The Pharmaceutical Journal* 1988; 241: 313-314.

9. Harding G, Taylor KMG. Pharmaceutical services and interprofessional communication in health centre pharmacies. *The Pharmaceutical Journal* 1989; 242: 21-22.

10. Harding G, Taylor KMG. The interface between pharmacists and general practitioners in English health centres. *The Pharmaceutical Journal* 1989; 242: 549-550.

11. Harding G, Taylor KMG. Professional relationships between general practitioners and pharmacists in health centres. *British Journal of General Practice* 1990; 40: 464-466.

12. Jefferys M, Sachs H. *Rethinking General Practice.* London: Tavistock; 1983.

13. Larkin G. *Occupational Monopoly and Modern Medicine.* London: Tavistock; 1983.

14. Bruce N. *Teamwork for Preventive Care.* London; Churchill Livingstone; 1980.

15. Campbell-Heider N, Pollock D. Barriers to physician-nurse collegiality: an anthropological perspective. *Social Science and Medicine* 1987; 25: 421-425.

16. Freidson E. *The Profession of Medicine: a Study of the Application of Medical Knowledge.* New York: Dodd Mead; 1970.

17. Armstrong D. The emancipation of biographical medicine *Social Science and Medicine* 1979; 13A 1-8.

18. Turner BS. *Medical Power and Social Knowledge.* London: Sage; 1987 p.145.

19. Williamson RE, Kabat HF. Pharmacist-physician drug communications. *Journal of the American Pharmaceutical Association* 1971; NS11: 164-167.

20. Smith GH, Sorby DL, Sharp LJ. Physicians' attitudes toward drug information resources. *American Journal of Hospital Pharmacy* 1975; 32: 19-25.

21. Ortiz M, Walker W-L, Thomas R. Physicians – friend or foe? *Journal of Social and Administrative Pharmacy* 1989; 6: 59-68.

22. Van de Poel G, Bruijnzeels MA, Van der Does J, Lubsen J. A way of achieving more rational drug prescribing? *International Journal of Pharmacy Practice* 1991; 1: 45-48.

CHAPTER SIX

THE PHARMACIST AND PRIMARY CARE: RESPONDING TO THE NEEDS OF MOTHERS WITH YOUNG CHILDREN

Sarah Cunningham-Burley

INTRODUCTION

Decision making over matters of health and illness is difficult and complex. Signs and symptoms have to be recognised and interpreted, by the sufferer, or his or her carer, by doctors and others who may form part of a network of advice. Decisions have to be made over how serious the symptoms are, and what, if anything, should be done about them. Any service or contribution which makes this decision-making process easier, with successful and satisfactory health outcomes, must be sought and welcomed. This presents a challenge to health care providers, and one community pharmacy is especially well placed to meet.

In order to make an effective contribution to the health care needs of the population, pharmacists will need to understand the place they are accorded by the population in their repertoire of responses to illness. The beliefs and practices of those who may come to a pharmacist to ask for advice, to buy over-the-counter medicines, or to collect a prescription are the important context within which community pharmacy operates. This chapter will examine some of these beliefs and practices in relation to how mothers deal with their children's illnesses: and focus on the role of the pharmacist within their responses to actual or potential illness.

THE STUDY AND ITS METHODS

The study on which this chapter is based aimed to investigate the everyday context of children's minor illnesses, focusing on the mothers' perspectives. The study explored how symptoms were recognised and managed by the mothers, and elicited their norms of help-seeking behaviour. We wanted to find out as much as possible about mothers' perceptions of health and illness, and their decision-making behaviour.[1] The study utilised qualitative, sociological techniques involving in-depth interviewing. This method is informal and unstructured, with data in the form of long interviews. This enables the subject or respondent to talk about his or her own ideas, attitudes and behaviours in their own words.

The researcher does not define what is important.[2] Such qualitative methods have been found to be particularly appropriate to understanding women's experiences, and provide a non-threatening environment that encourages the development of rapport between the researcher and researched.[3,4] The in-depth interviews thus elucidated the mothers' perspectives on health and illness. The interviews were based around a topic guide developed from pilot work. A wide range of issues were covered, and the women were encouraged to talk about what was important and relevant to them, while keeping the focus on minor or everyday illness as far as possible.

The women participating in the study were also asked to complete a health diary, so that day-to-day information on illness behaviour could be collected. The diaries thus provided a useful record of what the mothers did to monitor and attend to their children's health and well-being. The mothers were simply asked to note down if they had noticed anything in their children that day, and whether any form of action had been taken (for example a visit to a doctor).

A total of 54 women, with at least one child under the age of 5, were interviewed. All but one were married, and the median age was 28 years. A further six women were interviewed for the pilot study. All but two of the women contacted agreed to participate in the study. The interviews were all conducted by myself, and were tape recorded and transcribed in order to provide a full, written version of the data. A total of 42 health diaries were completed, totalling 927 days when information was collected. The study was carried out between 1983 and 1985, in a new town in Scotland. The data were analysed qualitatively,[5] which means the data were searched for themes and concepts to be drawn from the mothers' own words. Some of these are considered below.

RESULTS AND DISCUSSION

Three areas on which data were collected will be discussed in this section: firstly the way in which mothers recognised illness in their children is discussed. This forms the backdrop to subsequent help-seeking behaviour, and provides an understanding of the cultural context of illness behaviour.[6] Secondly, how mothers responded to symptoms will be examined. The third focus is specifically on the mothers' use of pharmacists, as a particular part of their repertoire of responses to their children's minor illnesses.

Recognising When a Child May Be Ill

Normality
Mothers (usually it is the mother) have to deal with all the ups and downs in their children's health, and make a welter of mundane observations and minor decisions regarding their childrens' well-being. This is often an unrecognised skill, but one which the mothers in this study were well aware they possessed:

> R. 35 'It's a funny thing with mothers – you can tell when they're [the children] are no' well'.*

Mothers were able to notice any deviations from normality in their children. Normality then, is an important concept in the culture of illness in families with young children.[7] Health and illness are related to normality in a variety of ways, and because of this relationship mothers were alert to deviations from the normal. Their ability to recognise what might be unusual was borne from the accumulated experience of their own child. What might be normal for one child, might indeed be unusual in another, as the following example indicates:

> SCB: 'What sort of things do you normally look out for then if you think they are sickening for something?'

> R17: 'Well, in the case of these two, if they do start to cry a bit more than normal...Both of them are not cry babies unless its really something'.

> R50: '...you get signs, and all the kids are different. If she is not really well, she stops eating'.

The mothers' recognition of illness and symptoms also appeared to be embedded in a common sense knowledge about what was normal and acceptable, for example for different children at different developmental stages. Normality could be interpreted as a yardstick that operated in a variety of ways: as a measure of whether or not the child was 'ill' with the condition, for example a cough, whether the child was sickening for something, was experiencing normal illness, or was experiencing illness normally. This provides some understanding of how mothers think about illness.

Changes in Behaviour
Behavioural changes were very important in the process of recognising illness, instead of, or in addition to physical symptoms such as a runny nose or stomach ache. These were built on the concept of normality. The mothers monitored their children closely. From the health diaries, something was noticed about a child on 49% of all the diary days. Physical symptoms were noted on 311 occasions,

---

* The quotes are drawn from the interviews and serve to illustrate the themes and concepts being discussed. The number (R35 etc.) simply refers to the respondent

with cough, runny nose, cuts and bruises being the most common. Behavioural changes were recorded 315 times, with changes in sleep patterns figuring prominently. Changes in mood, and in eating behaviour were also noted. These all seemed important because the child was not his or her normal self, illness could be present or healthy development might be jeopardised.

Deviation from normal behaviour could be perceived in any of four ways. Firstly, it could be seen as a precursor to illness:

> R12: 'But you ken when he's no well when he doesnae want sweeties and crisps, that's a sure sign there is something wrong with him'.

Secondly, it could be a result of illness, making the illness more of a concern:

> R33: 'I mean he couldn't sleep at night for this cough'.

Thirdly, it could be an illness or problem in itself:

> R41: 'She has been really good, I have not really had any bother, apart from not sleeping. That was a big problem at the time'.

Lastly, it could be a problem for the family:

> R50: 'It got to the stage that my husband was coming out of work at tea time and I was going to bed until he was ready for bed because it was the only way I was getting sleep'.

Behavioural changes here were not simply interpreted as clues to an underlying problem. Although they were sometimes interpreted as a symptom of illness, their relationship to health and illness was more complicated.

Responding to Symptoms

As noted above, mothers recognised many small changes in their children, offering careful monitoring on a day to day basis. Many of these changes did not result in any action being taken, except watching and waiting. Thus, many things noted in children that may be seen as a possible precursor to illness in fact revert back to normal without any further developments. As noted above, from the health diaries it was found that something was noted in the children on 49% of days, but action was only taken on 65% of these days.[7] Indeed, other studies have shown that most illness in the community does not come to the attention of any health professional, whether a health visitor, general practitioner or a community pharmacist.[8]

On those days when some kind of action was taken, the responses fell into three main categories.

a. Home Nursing and Remedies
Home nursing was a common response, mentioned 100 times in the diaries.

Dealing with cuts and grazes, providing hot drinks, encouraging a child to rest or to eat, and making a child with symptoms comfortable were all mentioned. 'Traditional remedies', such as poultices and herb teas, did not form a large part of the mothers' repertoire of action, and were only mentioned by a few.

b. Over-the-Counter Remedies
Providing over-the-counter remedies, was the commonest response to childrens' symptoms. These were mentioned 181 times in the diaries. Analgesics and bottles of cough medicine were the most frequently mentioned medicines. From this data, and from the interview data, it was found that mothers would make every effort to treat their child themselves, even though they may be sceptical about the efficacy of some over-the-counter medicines. A typical response was:

> R36: 'I'll just use....a cough bottle, if they have got a cough at night and they can't get to sleep. I don't know if it is more psychological, but I give them a spoonful and it's OK. But like most colds they have got to run their course'.

c. Professional Help
The health diaries provided data on when the mothers contacted the doctor, or other health centre staff. This did not include the pharmacists who operated without the health centre setting in the study. Professional contact was the least common response, mentioned only 33 times. Advice of a doctor was sought if the symptoms did not clear up, worsened, or if the mother felt the child required immediate attention. An example from the interviews illustrates this process:

> R17: 'If it didn't clear up, I would go to the doctor, but I like to try and fix them up myself first'.

Contact with health professionals at the health centre (usually the general practitioner) represented only 11% of all days when action was taken. The mothers said that they did not want to appear to be 'bothering the doctor'[9] and expressed reluctance about contacting a doctor over what might be purely a trivial condition. The overwhelming response to a child's symptoms was some form of self-care.

This brief account of the mothers' perspectives on health and illness in their children highlights the potential role of a community pharmacist. Self-care, especially in the form of over-the-counter medicines was an important response to symptoms. Children experience many changes which might indicate illness, and mothers may need advice and reassurance, while feeling that the doctor may not be the most appropriate person to go to. The next section examines the mothers' use of pharmacists.

USE OF THE PHARMACIST

Although it was clear from the data that the mothers in the study did not often use the doctor, in response to symptoms in their children, they did discuss their use of the pharmacist (or chemist) in the in-depth interviews. Since self-care in the form of over-the-counter medicines was important, then it is not surprising that the mothers had considerable contact with pharmacies and pharmacists or their assistants. Also, although the mothers developed a range of responses to their children's illnesses, and had considerable skills in recognising symptoms and changes, they still had to make frequent and difficult decisions: what action to take; what was serious and what was trivial. We also found that the mothers were worried about bothering the doctor, and did not want to be seen to be wasting his or her time. These three points are illustrated in the following interview excerpt:

> R27: 'But at my own expense I would go to the chemist and say "Look, so and so has got this, what do you recommend?" And I know I can get free prescriptions for the children but I don't like wasting the doctor's time'.

Four main themes describe the role pharmacists played in the repertoire of lay response to children's symptoms. These will be examined below.

a. Purchasing Over-The-Counter Medicines

As noted above, most mothers used proprietary medicines at some point. Their views about these varied. A very few did not use them, and would only use something prescribed by a doctor. Some found particular brands especially helpful, and would have a favourite bottle (often recommended by a chemist), while others would try different items with varying success. Most of the mothers attempted to care for their children themselves. Many mothers said that they felt they had to do something, or buy something for their children to relieve their symptoms. Importantly, they felt that they were being good mothers by responding actively to the situation. The cost of proprietary medicines was also discussed by the mothers. There was an underlying tension in some of the families' use of doctors or chemists (the mothers tended to refer to pharmacists as chemists) for medicines which could be obtained free on prescription, but there were many occasions when, taking the financial cost into consideration, the mothers would go to the chemist, as the following example illustrates:

> R42: '...it was the chemist that told me to get them. I mean they are quite expensive but I don't bother, I'd rather that than go to the doctor. I mean I think I would go to the doctor if they were really ill or anything'.

The chemist often provided a means of doing something about children's symptoms without having to resort to a general practitioner. While some of the mothers used chemists for advice on treatment, many had only minimal contact, perhaps not even with the pharmacist him or herself, when buying medicines.

b. A Stepping Stone to the Doctor
Pharmacists may provide the first point of contact for advice and treatment of children's minor conditions. This first step might lead on to the doctors, if the condition did not clear up, or if the pharmacist recommended that a consultation with a general practitioner was sought. For example, in response to a question asking if she found the pharmacist helpful, a mother replied:

> R27: 'Yes, they'll either say "Try this" but you know yourself they are not very ill, there's not much point in bothering the doctor, or "try this", and after a day or two take them to the doctor, if things don't improve'.

c. An Alternative to the Doctor
Not all visits to the pharmacist were stepping stones to the doctor; they were often the only action taken in response to a child's symptoms. For the mothers in this study such visits were often an alternative to the doctor, providing a service which meant that they did not have to bother the doctor at all. As one mother said of a pharmacist:

> R23: 'They'll give you an idea what's wrong with them. Do the doctors out of a job! But I would rather take my child there if it just something they could give a bottle for, and he would get better, rather than take him to the doctor, and waste his time'.

The advantages of the community pharmacist is that they are readily accessible to the public, and their advice is considered appropriate for dealing with minor illnesses in children. It may be what the doctor would suggest anyway:

> R42: 'I would go and get Actifed or something because if I go to the doctor that's what he would probably give me initially anyway unless she had it for two or three weeks and couldn't shift it'.*

d. Better than the Doctor
A few of the mothers said that they found the pharmacist better than the doctor, and felt his or her advice and recommendations more appropriate. They may have been displeased with the treatment of a doctor. The pharmacist may be seen as responding to mothers' concerns, and thus fit in to the mothers' own understandings and needs.

> R35: 'He (the doctor) said just to continue with the Actifed* and it still wasn't clearing up, so I went into a chemist in the city one Saturday, and I spoke to the pharmacist, and she stood and listened – a young lassie, but

---

* This study was conducted prior to the introduction of the limited list which limited the prescribing of many medicines including proprietary cough medicines such as Actifed.

she was awfully nice – she stood and she listened and she asked you questions, and she said well I think with the type of cough they've got they've been on Actifed too long, and it's not taking any effect. It's for the wrong sort of cough. So she made me up a bottle of cough medicine and she says, "But it's dear, you usually only get this on prescription. It'll cost you about a pound". And it did. I said 'I'm no fussy hen, so long as it helps my bairns'.''

IMPLICATIONS FOR CURRENT AND FUTURE PHARMACY PRACTICE

This study has shown the importance of pharmacists within the range of responses mothers had to minor illness and symptoms in their children. Blaxter and Paterson[10] have also noted that help-seeking and lay advice may be as important as consultation with doctors. In their three generational study of health attitudes and behaviour, Blaxter and Paterson found that the mothers in their study reported more use of chemists for advice than the grandmothers, but that the latter said that they had used chemists when they were younger. The marked difference between the generations as far as home care was concerned was an increase in the use of proprietary medicine amongst the mothers, with less use of 'home remedies' compared to the older generation.

It is clear that pharmacists or 'chemists' and proprietary medicines, both separately and together, play a significant part in lay health care. The mothers of young children in the study reported here, used chemists in a variety of ways. They had different attitudes to pharmacists' role, and also to the use and purchase of proprietary medicines. The majority of the mothers did purchase medicines at some time, and this alone has implications for the role of pharmacists as educators, advice givers or information disseminators. There is considerable scope for developing existing contacts between the pharmacist and mothers and in promoting good self care. The pharmacist may be able to provide advice on home nursing, and provide other health related advice.

Briefly, the pharmacist was used as advice giver (providing 'differential diagnosis') and reassurer. Their role was sometimes as a stepping stone to a doctor, or sometimes as an alternative to the doctor (and sometimes considered better than the doctor). Also, the chemist was used to purchase proprietary medicines, and contact may only be fleeting. Underlying the mothers' use of chemists seemed to be a concern not to bother the doctor with trivial conditions. Chemists seemed to be in a unique position, being able to assist mothers in making their own decisions about responding to their children's health problems. The chemist, as advice giver and vendor of proprietary medicines, often enabled mothers to do something for their child without going to the doctor.

It would seem that pharmacists do provide a valuable service to many mothers with young children. They are flexible and informal, and enable mothers to cope with a symptomatic child who does not need the attention of a doctor. They provide an external source of advice, and provide an important link between lay and professional responses to illness. They can potentially enhance mothers' own competencies.

This intermediary position as someone in between lay and medical responses to illness reflects some ambiguity in the role of community pharmacist.[11] They may rest uneasily between being part of the primary care team – that is, providing professional health care, along with general practitioners, health visitors and nurses – and being part of a lay health network, being used by the public to respond to their health needs without resort to health professions. This ambiguity is also present in any historical analysis of the pharmacy profession, and it is also evident in an analysis of the relationship between pharmacy and the medical profession, whose roles at a local level may overlap and merge (see Britten, Chapter 4).[12] Woodward[13] has noted that the apothecaries of the past gradually extended their function from keeping chemists' shops to compounding prescriptions and prescribing for and treating patients in their own homes. They had some functions similar to that of the general practitioner today. Apothecaries, and now chemists, had and have a potentially competitive relationship with physicians because their skills and functions can overlap. Yet, it is precisely this potential overlap which is the pharmacists strength. As the Nuffield Report suggests, "...if members of the public decide, for whatever reason, that they would rather in any particular instance call on a pharmacist than visit their doctor, the pharmacist must be ready and equipped to respond".[14] There have been calls to extend the role of the community pharmacist,[15] and from the mothers' accounts it would seem that there is scope for expansion of the role of the pharmacist. Measures to indicate to the public what the pharmacist's role and skills are, would be useful. Pharmacists could reinforce mothers' abilities to cope with minor illnesses in their children, thus improving self-esteem. As mothers were concerned with deviations from the normal, and with their child's health development, pharmacists could advise appropriately about what is normal, as well as offering treatment for self-limiting episodes. At a local and national level co-operation between community pharmacists and general practitioners could avert any conflict in roles, instead providing a comprehensive service which meets the needs of those caring for young children.

ACKNOWLEDGEMENT

This study was funded by the Scottish Home and Health Department and conducted within the Department of Community Medicine (now Public Health Sciences), University of Edinburgh with Dr Una Maclean and Dr Sandy Irvine.

REFERENCES

1. Cunningham-Burley S, Irvine S. And have you done anything so far: An examination of lay treatment of children's symptoms. *British Medical Journal* 1987; 295: 700-702.
2. Lofland J, Lofland L. *Analyzing Social Settings*. California: Wadsworth Publishing Company; 1984.
3. Oakley A. Interviewing women: A contradiction in terms. In: Roberts H. ed. *Doing Feminist Research*. London: Routledge and Kegan Paul; 1981.
4. Graham H. Surveying through stores. In: Bell C, Roberts H. eds. *Social Researching, Politics, Problems and Practice*. London: Routledge and Kegan Paul; 1984.
5. Strauss A, Corbin J. *Basics of Qualitative Research*. London: Sage Publications; 1990.
6. Cunningham-Burley S. Mothers' beliefs about and perceptions of their children's illnesses. In: Cunningham-Burley S, McKeganey N. eds. *Readings in Medical Sociology*. London: Routledge; 1990.
7. Irvine S, Cunningham-Burley S. Mothers' concepts of normality, behavioural change and illness in their children. *British Journal of General Practice* 1991; 41: 371-374.
8. Hannay D. *The Symptom Iceberg; a study of community health*. London: Routledge and Kegan Paul; 1979.
9. Cunningham-Burley S, Maclean U. Dealing with Children's Illnesses: Mothers' dilemmas. In: Wyke S, Hewison J. eds. *Child Health Matters*. Milton Keynes: Open University Press; 1991.
10. Blaxter M, Paterson E. *Mothers and Daughters: A Three Generational Study of Health Attitudes and Behaviour*. London: Routledge and Kegan Paul; 1982.
11. Cunningham-Burley S, Maclean U. The Role of the Chemist in Primary Health Care for Children with Minor Complaints. *Social Science and Medicine* 1987; 24: 371-377.
12. Eaton G, Webb B. Boundary encroachment: pharmacists in the clinical setting. *Sociology of Health and Illness* 1979; 1: 69-89.
13. Woodward J. *To Do the Sick No Harm*. London: Routledge and Kegan Paul; 1974.
14. Nuffield Committee of Inquiry into Pharmacy. *Pharmacy: a Report to the Nuffield Foundation*. London: Nuffield Foundation; 1986.
15. Rawlins MD. Extending the role of the community pharmacist. *British Medical Journal* 1991; 302: 427-428.

CHAPTER SEVEN

PRIMARY CARE CONSULTATIONS IN COMMUNITY PHARMACY

Felicity Smith

INTRODUCTION

Pharmacists have a long history as health advisors to the public. Trease[1] traces the development of the profession from spicers (the earliest traders of drugs and spices) of the 12th century, through spicer-apothecaries of the later middle ages to druggists, dispensing chemists and apothecaries of the 17th, 18th and 19th centuries. In the 16th and 17th century when there were few physicians, the apothecaries would treat their clients' ailments; physicians being employed only by the gentry or in cases of severe illness.[2]

In Britain the Pharmaceutical Society was formed in 1841 comprising druggists (purely retailers or suppliers of medicines), dispensing chemists and apothecaries (both of whom counter prescribed, made up their own medical preparations and carried out minor surgical operations such as drawing teeth, lancing boils or bandaging wounds in their shops).[3] Sharp[4] writing about his father's pharmacy business of the early 20th century describes how he gained an "impressive reputation for curing ills". He asserts that counter-prescribing was important to most pharmacies, especially in the poorer areas as there was no National Health Service and people could not afford to see a doctor.

During the 20th century there have been vast developments in health care technology and changes in health care delivery, with corresponding implications for the professional roles of all health care personnel. The British Government, as many governments throughout the world, acknowledges the importance of these developments believing that increased emphasis on primary care and health promotion is the most effective strategy for securing greatest improvements in the health status of the population[5].

Despite many changes in the structure and delivery of health care services the traditional role of pharmacists as counter-prescribers for minor ailments has continued and its development is encouraged both within the profession and by the Government.

This chapter will review the current contribution made by pharmacists to primary health care in dealing with minor illness in the community, and will consider the developments necessary to ensure that this function is carried out effectively and in line with planned changes in health care delivery.

PHARMACISTS AND MINOR AILMENTS

Although the pharmacist's role in responding to clients who present with minor ailments is longstanding and well-recognised, formal investigations of the extent and quality of this role had not been performed until recently. From around the late 1970s, surveys investigating symptoms presented to community pharmacists have been conducted.[6-13] These surveys have found the average pharmacist in Britain advises around 10 clients a day on minor ailments: country-wide this corresponds to over 100,000 consultations per day or 30 million in a year. The range of symptoms uncovered in many of these studies will be familiar to most community pharmacists. Most cases can be categorised into a few broad groups (Figure 1), in particular upper respiratory, skin and gastrointestinal symptoms.

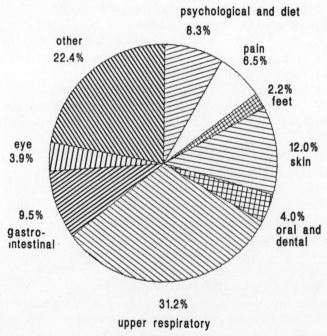

Figure 1: Symptoms presented to pharmacists: main categories (n=947). From reference 14.

However, more detailed examination of symptoms presented to pharmacists shows that these broad categorisations conceal a wide range of presentations requiring different responses from, and skills of, the pharmacist. For example "skin symptoms" include short-term, self-limiting problems and chronic problems in which there may be a more serious underlying disease (Figure 2). If a product is supplied, it may be a palliative or curative remedy, or first aid. When advising, it may be appropriate for the pharmacist to consider possible underlying causes and suggest ways of preventing recurrence. Some of these skin symptoms although possibly considered by pharmacists to be minor, have psychological implications, requiring an awareness and sensitivity by the pharmacist.

It may be argued that all cases presented to pharmacists will have a psychological and social component which the pharmacist must acknowledge in the consultation to ensure that the advice given is appropriate to the client's needs. However, there are some symptoms that may be considered as primarily psychological in nature. For example, a study of consultations between London pharmacists and clients included a discussion following a recent bereavement, general well-being, anxiety, insomnia and weight problems[14].

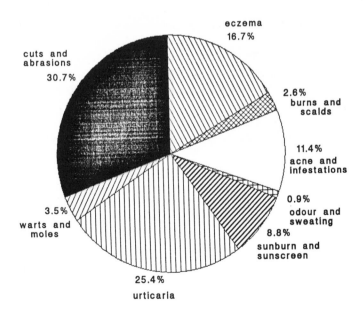

Figure 2: Skin symptoms and conditions presented to pharmacists (n=114). From reference 14.

Some clients may request over-the-counter products that interact with their prescribed medication[15], or be otherwise contraindicated; this presents a further consideration for pharmacists in ensuring the safe management of minor illness. Thus as well as requiring a broad clinical and pharmaceutical knowledge and skills to respond to the wide range of symptoms presented, pharmacists also require good communication skills and an awareness of psychological and social aspects of health and ill-health. If their advisory role is to be valued, pharmacists need to ensure a high quality of service. In recent years there have been several investigations into the quality of advice given by pharmacists.[16-28] These studies frequently involve a researcher posing as a client and presenting at several pharmacies with a predetermined case-history. Following each visit the researcher records certain details of the pharmacist's response. Such investigations have clear limitations; they cannot provide a comprehensive assessment of the quality of the pharmacist's advisory role, as they focus on particular symptoms and scenarios, noting whether specific questions were asked or items of advice were given in these cases. Nor do they provide an indication of how pharmacists deal with the wide range of presentations, clients and problems that are part of their daily practice.

On the whole, pharmacists have been found to be readily available to clients requesting advice, but frequently these studies have highlighted deficiencies in the questions asked by pharmacists; relevant and important details not being established, and sometimes the most appropriate advice not being supplied. For example, despite publicity on the cross-sensitivity between aspirin and ibuprofen, many pharmacists supplied an ibuprofen product to "clients" presenting with muscular symptoms and sensitivity to aspirin.[19]

In another study, only 28% of pharmacists who were presented with "cases" of dysmenorrhoea were considered to have asked the most important questions, ie. those concerning duration, nature, timing, other medicines and disease states.[28] In a study investigating the responses of pharmacists to clients with coughs it was found that in only a quarter of cases was the duration of symptoms established, accompanying symptoms were discussed in only half the consultations and in only five of the 92 cases was the issue of other medication being taken raised.[27] Whilst, in response to requests for advice on vitamins, pharmacists were considered to ask too few questions: this may lead to inappropriate supply.[21] Concern was also expressed about the extent to which responding to symptoms is left to counter-assistants, an issue of continuing concern.[18,22] Following interviews with community pharmacists, in which they were questioned about responding to ocular symptoms, researchers were critical of the responses; many pharmacists reported that they had received no relevant training.[26]

The studies which have received the widest publicity are those of the Consumers' Association.[16,20,23] These have focused on various issues, such as whether the pharmacist recommended the cheapest suitable product and the availability of a private area for the consultation. In their most recent investigation they criticised pharmacists for not identifying potentially serious symptoms and offering appropriate referral advice. These studies have generally met with criticism on methodological grounds though they have also highlighted some deficiencies in the quality of advice. In the 1991 Consumers' Association survey, two-thirds of the pharmacists recommended oral rehydration therapy, (considered the treatment of choice for children with diarrhoea), for a two-year-old child with diarrhoea. In a similar study, oral rehydration therapy was recommended in only 30% of cases. Although in the latter study, the small sample size (only 10 pharmacists) renders the validity and generalisability of the results as questionable, this study attracted wide publicity.[24] In a further study in which genuine consultations between pharmacists and members of the public were recorded, eight of the 711 consultations concerned young children with diarrhoea. A product was recommended and sold by six of these pharmacists and in all cases this was oral rehydration therapy.[25] Variations in the findings of these studies may be due to real variation (eg regional), the methods selected for the study and/or sample size.

Methodological Issues

It can be argued that the cases presented to pharmacists by researchers posing as clients may not represent types of consultations with which pharmacists are confronted in their daily practice. Assessment of pharmacists' responses to real consultations between pharmacists and clients overcomes this problem, but the collection of detailed data on large numbers of consultations between pharmacists and members of the public presents many practical problems. Consultations may be few or many and occur any time of the day.

Covert research produces a response from the pharmacist that is unbiased in that pharmacists are unaware of the study and therefore unable to modify their responses, but this method depends on the ability of the researcher to simulate a real client, (this issue was addressed in a study of pharmacists' management of dysmenorrhoea[28]). The ethics of covert research methods, within pharmacy have also been questioned.[29] Such methods cannot be used when the informed consent of the subjects is required.

In assessing the quality of care the most appropriate method to be employed will depend on the objectives of the study. The results must be interpreted accordingly: for instance if a "non-covert" method is used, awareness of a study would not affect the participants' knowledge of what constitutes good practice, but may affect the extent to which they follow this.

Variation in clinical judgement reflecting differing preferences of individual practitioners regarding good practice is widely acknowledged. Attempts have been made to overcome this subjectivity.[30] However, in assessing the quality of care a decision has to be made about whose criteria to use. Consumers, individual practitioners and each professional group may have different perspectives on what they believe to comprise appropriate care. Every consultation is a unique encounter between the client and the professional. Reliable and valid methods for the assessment of quality in health care are rapidly developing. However, irrespective of the method used to assess the quality of pharmacist's responses to symptoms, genuine causes for concern have been identified which must be confronted.

PRIMARY CARE CONSULTATIONS AND HEALTH PROMOTION

The most common causes of mortality in Britain, including premature death, are diseases for which risk factors (especially smoking, poor diet, alcohol and lack of exercise) have been identified. Most notably these include cardiovascular disease (to which 46% of deaths in 1991 were attributed), cancers (25%) and respiratory disease (11%).[31] The recent Government White Paper "Health of the Nation"[5] sets out a strategy for health. Disease prevention and health promotion are emphasised as ways in which improvements in the health status of the population can be secured. The document focuses on priority areas with targets relating to the year 2000 that include coronary heart disease, strokes and cancers. These areas were selected because of the scope for prevention of disease and death.

Inequalities in health status of different social groups in Britain are well-recognised.[32,33] Moreover, it is those people who enjoy better general health who are more likely to act upon health promotion messages. This was reflected in the relative decline in smoking among different socio-economic groups throughout the 1980s.[33] A similar trend is still apparent: examination of the clientele of well-women and well-men clinics in primary care in recent years has found the preferential uptake of services by people of higher health status, sometimes termed "the worried well".[34] If health promotion is to be an effective strategy for health care delivery the problem of getting the messages to people who could benefit the most needs to be addressed.

A broad cross-section of the population use pharmacies. Community pharmacists are being encouraged by their professional body, the Royal Pharmaceutical Society, to become more active in promoting health; a development that has been endorsed in an independent inquiry into pharmacy conducted by the Nuffield Foundation,[35] and in a Government White Paper "Promoting Better Health".[36]

Few studies into the advisory role of the pharmacist have concentrated on the health promotion input. One study in which pharmacists kept diaries of requests for advice from clients, found that most symptom-related enquiries did not lead on to a discussion about general health.[12]

There is now a substantial body of literature on concepts, approaches and values of health promotion. Beattie summarising these, distinguishes individual approaches (responding to the needs of individuals) and collective approaches (economic, environmental and health policy making; and community projects)[37]. The health promotion role that can be part of the daily practice of the community pharmacist is based on the provision of personal health care services to individuals who visit the pharmacy (though there may also be occasions for community pharmacy to participate in, or be a focus for, a community health promotion programme, particularly when the pharmacy is an integrated part of the community).

The "individual approach" involves, first, the giving of information appropriate for the presenting symptom, for example informing a client on the link between smoking and cough. This requires that pharmacists can identify possible underlying causes of symptoms and are prepared to discuss them. Secondly it involves helping individuals to feel in control of, take responsibility for, or manage their situation (for example helping the individual cope with health related problems). This requires a listening, responding and supporting approach where the pharmacist creates an atmosphere in which clients can express their concerns, the pharmacist being prepared to listen, acknowledge and constructively respond to these concerns. Thus pharmacists need good communication skills: questioning (using open and closed questions) in a way that elicits the relevant information from clients, time to listen and pay attention to detail in the clients' requests and responses. Such an approach may also facilitate the discernment of "hidden agendas" (concerns that clients are hesitant to raise). (See also chapter 9).

The "individual approach" acknowledges that individuals have a fundamental role in maintaining their health status and that the relationship between the client and the health care professional should be a partnership, both working with the same ultimate aim. Models of professional-client interaction have been developed according to the degree of involvement of both parties. At one extreme the consultation may be dominated by the professional with the client remaining passive, at the other, a situation in which both parties actively participate in the decision-making process.[38] Korsch et al, in a study of doctor-patient communication found that when individuals had a greater participation in the consultation they were more likely to be satisfied with it, and that satisfied clients were more likely to have followed advice.[39]

Pharmacies are pre-eminently a source of medication. Knowledge of products and their uses is recognised as an area of pharmacists' particular expertise.

However, health promotion requires that in responding to symptoms, the consultation includes some focus on the presentation and nature of the symptoms, including an exploration of possible causes, contributory factors, and their implications for the daily lives of the clients. Thus a consultation that is merely confined to a discussion and/or supply of available products will not promote opportunities for health promotion ideas.

The following cases are transcriptions of consultations between pharmacists (P) and clients (C) in community pharmacies. These illustrate some characteristics of aspects of consultations (cases reproduced with permission, from reference 40).

Case one:

In this example the pharmacist focused his/her information around products:

C: Is Metatone an iron tonic?
P: No, not iron. We do have iron preparations.
C: I feel kind of exhausted.
P: We've got iron tablets.
C: I just want some energy.
P: Well, if you want iron on it's own . . .

The pharmacist did not respond to information from the client about their symptoms, though the client attempted to raise these issues more than once. Later in the same consultation, when the pharmacist asked the client one question about their appetite this seemed to be prompted by, and geared to, the selection of a product:

P: ...this has phosphate in it which helps your appetite. Are you eating well?
C: Yes.
P: Then I reckon an iron tonic.

In other cases (eg two and three below) the pharmacist did question the appropriateness of the products requested by the client:

Case two:

C: Do you have Calcium and Vitamin D tablets?
P: Do you need calcium? Do you not drink milk, eat cheese, yoghurt . . . ?

Case three:

C: I want some vitamins.
P: Why do you think you need vitamins?

Case four:

This consultation followed a request from an elderly client for a particular tonic. The pharmacist took the opportunity to explore the symptoms and review the client's health status to ensure that the most appropriate care was recommended:

P: Is it for you?
C: Yes.
P: Do you eat well?
C: Erm, not particularly, no .
P: Do you feel low or . . .?
C: Yes. I haven't got any energy, it took me all my time to walk round here. I know I'm old but I thought there might be something to help me.
P: Are you having any treatment from the doctor?
C: No, no
P: How about your skin, do you have any problems or anything?
C: No, nothing like that.

The pharmacist selected a multivitamin preparation, which he explained may help the client as she isn't eating particularly well. He explained dosing regimes, and ensured that she was seeing her doctor regularly to have her blood pressure checked.

A systematic pattern of domination by either the pharmacist or the client was not a feature of these consultations, in the way that is usual in medical consultations.[41] This probably reflects the pharmacist-client relationship as more equal; the client is unlikely to feel under an obligation to accept advice. In terms of the delivery of health promotion in community pharmacies, this would be expected to be advantageous in that clients may feel more relaxed and able to raise their concerns, request clarification of advice or challenge recommendations. Professional domination is possibly more likely to occur with poorer socio-economic groups.[41]

Pharmacists' clients comprise many different social, cultural and ethnic groups reflecting society. Medical and health practices of different cultural groups and the implications for health care personnel have been explored.[42-44] It is important that practitioners have an awareness of the variation in perceptions of health, need and use of services by different groups if an appropriate and relevant service is to be provided.

Researchers in a Bradford pharmacy[45] (an area with a large Asian population) observed that a smaller proportion of Asians entering the pharmacy sought the advice of the pharmacist, or purchased over-the-counter remedies compared with the indigenous population. This study involved only one pharmacy and possibly the behaviour of a single coherent ethnic minority group. A study in Nottingham[46] found Asian mothers less likely to give their children over-the-counter medicines than the white indigenous mothers. While these results cannot be extrapolated to the diversity of cultural groups, they are examples of differing perspectives and practices in responding to health and illness in different cultural groups. Aslam and Healy[47] have pointed out that traditional Asian community doctors, known as Hakims, either prepare medicines themselves or have assistants who do not give advice. The concept of a pharmacist, with some medical knowledge, is not well accepted. The authors argue that as a result these Asian groups make scant use of pharmacy advisory services, instead visiting the general medical practitioner more frequently.

Apart from groups with particular cultural needs there are also diagnostic groups such as people with mental illness and learning difficulties who are increasingly being cared for in the community and thus more likely to come into contact with community pharmacy services. There will be as many different sorts of consultations as there are pharmacists, and there is no "blueprint" for a good consultation. However, it is important that practitioners develop their own style ensuring that it effectively and efficiently achieves the objectives of the consultation, promoting and pursuing opportunities for health promotion. Emphasis on health promotion is an explicit part of the Government's health policy priorities and endorsed by the health professions.

THE PRIMARY HEALTH CARE TEAM

Many studies have shown that culture, social networks and lay consultations, among other factors are important contributory factors in determining patterns of uptake of professional health care services.[48,49] Many cases of illness and disease are known not to reach the formal health sector, remaining untreated, and thus termed "unmet need".[50] However, many cases of "unmet need" may get as far as a pharmacy. One study found that for 79% of clients presenting symptoms to a pharmacist, this was their first (and may be their only) contact with the professional health care services.[51] Before presenting symptoms to a health care professional, advice from friends and relatives may be sought. This is called the "lay referral system" or "lay-referral network". If pharmacists acknowledge their position and take on the responsibility, they could serve as a link between the professional and lay referral networks. Clients have been shown to use pharmacists as both an alternative, and a stepping-stone, to the doctor or for supplementary advice.[52,53] (See also chapter 6).

Recent criticism of the practice of pharmacists by the Consumers' Association[23] focused on the failure of pharmacists to refer clients who, they considered, presented with potentially serious symptoms that required further investigation by a medical practitioner. Pharmacists in consultations with clients could play an important part in identifying such cases, offering referral advice that will benefit individual clients and promote an efficient and appropriate demand for health care services.

Although pharmacists are often viewed as working in relative isolation, their role in responding to symptoms will be in conjunction with other primary carers, notably general medical practitioners (to whom most referrals are made), district nurses and health visitors. The different primary care professionals inevitably share clients and deal with many similar types of problems. In a study of consultations in London pharmacies approximately one in seven clients was either directly referred (advised to see another health professional when possible) or conditionally referred (advised to seek further advice should the

Table 1: Number of conditional and direct referrals (n=716)
(adapted from reference 48).

Outcome	Number (%)
Client not referred	616 (86.0)
direct referral	*60 (8.4)
Conditional referral	^40 (5.6)

*In all but six of these cases the pharmacist gave advice about medication an/or symptoms in addition to advice to seek assistance from another practitioner.

^In all but one of these cases the pharmacist gave advice about medication and/or symptoms in addition to advice to seek assistance from another practitioner.

Table 2: Personnel to whom clients were referred
(reproduced with permission from reference 48).

	Number of Cases		
	conditional referral	direct referral	all
General medical practitioner	44	45	90
GMP or specialist		1	1
GMP or hospital		1	1
Accident and emergency dept		4	4
Hospital (OPD clinic)		2	2
Dentist	1	4	5
Chiropodist		2	2
Nurse		2	2
Health Visitor	1		1

symptoms not have cleared or subsided within a given period or with a particular medication) (Table 1).[54] Although most referrals were to general medical practitioners, a quarter of direct referrals was to other agencies (Table 2). There was wide variation in referral rates depending on the nature of the symptoms. Pharmacists referred 8% of clients with upper respiratory symptoms, 15% with skin and 17% with gastrointestinal symptoms. Pharmacists referred over half of the clients with ear symptoms and nearly a quarter of those with symptoms concerning the eye.

Pharmacists also receive requests for advice, a "second opinion," or clarification on medication or management of problems by other health care professionals. For example, a study of the consultations in London pharmacies included requests for advice on benziodiazepine withdrawal and a wish to discuss a referral by a medical practitioner to an alcohol clinic.[14]

Health Visitors and District Nurses

At present there is little documentation on relations between nurses and pharmacists. Work that has been conducted suggests that liaison is rather limited, the purpose of the vast majority of contacts being for the supply of particular products, although opportunities for wider collaboration are likely to exist.[55] Health visitors have a particular responsibility for the health care of young children. Approximately one-sixth of consultations in pharmacies concern children of which more than a quarter are under two years of age.[56] The frequency of such consultations in pharmacies may be affected by the fact that under the National Health Service children are entitled to free prescriptions. The problems commonly presented to pharmacists include coughs, colds, diarrhoea and vomiting, wind, feeding, nappy rash, teething, and hair infestation; matters on which health visitors also regularly advise.[56] Consultations concerning children were more likely to occur in pharmacies in residential areas than in the town/city centre pharmacies. This suggests that pharmacists, along with health visitors, offer a service to local children, with whom they may have a continuing relationship and provide on-going care.

Pharmacists, nurses, health visitors and general medical practitioners are all developing their roles in disease prevention and health promotion. Interprofessional collaboration would enable coordination of disease prevention and health promotion activities: when responding to the needs of individual clients and their minor ailments, when discussing general care such as feeding and teething, and when advising on public health issues such as immunization policies and dealing with hair infestation. The work of district nurses necessitates responding to needs of individual clients, in particular, elderly people with chronic illness, or returning home after surgery. Again pharmacists and nurses will share many clients. District nurses have an understanding of the health problems of their clients, pharmacists have a detailed knowledge of available medical products. Working together, they should be able to ensure that each client receives the most appropriate products. Pharmacists are also in a position to offer advice and support to the lay-carers. The introduction of nurse-prescribing should provide many more opportunities for collaboration. An independent prescribing role will confer more autonomous responsibility for patient care. In their management decisions, nurses will need to be aware of uses and contraindications of the drugs they are prescribing as well as other drugs which clients may be using concurrently.

IMPLICATIONS FOR THE FUTURE

Interprofessional awareness of each other's roles and practices, a sharing of expertise and co-ordination of advice will in the future enhance the effectiveness of the pharmacist's advisory role and promote a more efficient primary care service of benefit to the professions and the public. This is also promoted by the British Government as the most effective and efficient way forward for the delivery of primary care. Health promotion is an explicit part of the Government's health policy and has been widely endorsed by the health professions. A high quality service in this area requires the provision of a suitable environment as well as attention to the content and conduct of consultations.

The availability of private counselling areas within pharmacies has been a subject of discussion within the pharmaceutical profession for some time. A call for such areas in all community pharmacies was made by the President of the Pharmaceutical Society in 1983.[57] The issue has been the subject of a recent editorial and a special feature in *The Pharmaceutical Journal*.[58,59] Clients frequently wish to discuss problems of a personal nature with pharmacists. The lack of privacy may inhibit clients from bringing problems to pharmacists and/or pharmacists or clients raising relevant but sensitive issues during consultations. One study, for example, reported that 45.5% of clients questioned, claimed to have felt at sometime that there was insufficient privacy.[60] In a postal survey of residents in the Grampian region of Scotland, 54% of respondents wanted a private consultation area, the only facility requested by more people was a seated waiting area.[61] The lack of privacy for consultations has also been highlighted in other studies (including those of the Consumers' Association).[23,62] These findings suggest that if pharmacists are to develop a satisfactory service this issue should be addressed.

The provision of private areas brings practical problems such as availability of space and ensuring adequate supervision of supply of medicines. However, the provision of separate areas will assure clients that they have the undivided attention of the pharmacist, creating an atmosphere in which questions can be asked and clarification requested. Private areas will also show to clients the importance that the pharmaceutical profession attaches to the advisory role and the need for confidentiality.

In addition to considering physical structures which facilitate pharmacist-client communication and promote the role of the pharmacist as health advisor, the educational needs of pharmacists and future pharmacists also require consideration. Schools of pharmacy should ensure students acquire the necessary knowledge, skills and attitudes (see also Chapter 15). For instance pharmacists are not usually in a position to make a diagnosis. However, they need the skills and knowledge base to gather comprehensive information to enable them to make informed judgements. They also require an awareness of the implications of a problem so that the relevant information is obtained from the client. Pharmacists should be competent in providing clear instructions and explanations for a course of action, in terms of short and long-term management and respond fully to issues raised by clients. Pharmacists must be able to make appropriate choices of medication when counter-prescribing, whilst also being aware of underlying causes of ill health or contributory factors. They should be prepared to discuss these and other lifestyle issues, such as smoking and diet, and their implications for their clients' daily lives. Pharmacists need to be aware of other primary care services, possess clinical knowledge to enable them to recognise cases in which there may be more serious underlying disease so appropriate referral advice can be offered.

Pharmacists should be prepared to listen, to create an atmosphere and consulting style that permits clients to express their concerns, and respond to these constructively.

REFERENCES

1. Trease GE. *Pharmacy in History*. London: Balliere, Tindall and Cox; 1964.
2. Matthews LG. The spicers and apothecaries of Norwich. *The Pharmaceutical Journal* 1967; 198: 5-9.
3. Burnby JGL. A study of the English Apothecary from 1660 to 1760. *Medical History* Supplement No 3. London: Wellcome Institute for the History of Medicine; 1983.
4. Sharp LK. Prussic Acid, Patients and Professors. *The Pharmaceutical Journal* 1985; 235: 821-822.
5. Government White Paper. *Health of the Nation*. London: HMSO (Cmd 1986); 1992.
6. Whitfield M. The pharmacist's contribution to medical care. *Practitioner* 1968; 200: 434-8.
7. Bass M. The pharmacist as a provider of primary care. *Canadian Medical Association Journal* 1975; 12: 60-64.

8. Boylan LJ. Advisory role of the pharmacist. *The Pharmaceutical Journal* 1978; 221: 328.

9. Sharpe D. The pattern of over-the-counter prescribing. *Mims Magazine* 15 September 1979: 39-45.

10. Phelan MJ, Jepson MH. The advisory role of the general practice pharmacist. *The Pharmaceutical Journal* 1980; 223: 584.

11. D'Arcy PF, Irwin WG, Clarke D, Kerr J, Gorman W, O'Sullivan D. The Role of the General Practice Pharmacist in Primary Health Care. *The Pharmaceutical Journal* 1980; 223: 539-542.

12. Shafford A, Sharpe K. *The Pharmacist as a Health Educator.* Health Education Authority: London; 1988.

13. Smith FJ, Salkind MR. Presentation of Clinical Symptoms to Community Pharmacists in London. *Journal of Social and Administrative Pharmacy* 1990; 7: 221-224.

14. Smith FJ. The contribution of community pharmacists to primary health care in London. Unpublished PhD thesis, University of London, 1989.

15. Chua S-S, Benrimoj SI, Stewart K, Williams G. Usage of non-prescription medications by hypertensive patients. *Journal of Social and Administrative Pharmacy* 1991; 8: 33-45.

16. Edwards J, Attan J, Wilson A, White B, Herxheimer A. General practice pharmacists: how good is the advice they give patients? *The Pharmaceutical Journal* 1975; 218: 568.

17. Feehan HV. Study of pharmacists' counselling competency. *The Pharmaceutical Journal* 1980; 225: 172-173.

18. Hardistry B. Do assistants take the pharmacist's role in counter-prescribing? *Chemist and Druggist* 1982; 218: 804-808.

19. Morley A, Jepson MH. How pharmacists respond to symptoms. UK Clinical Pharmacy Association/May and Baker Community Pharmacy Award, 1984.

20. Consumers' Association. Advice Across the Chemist's Counter. *Which?* 1985; 8: 351-354.

21. Gill Y, Gill Z, Scully C. How community pharmacy staff manage recurrent mouth ulcers. *The Pharmaceutical Journal* 1988; 241: 82-83.

22. McGuinness ME, Rathbone MR, Trevean MA. Vitamins and minerals: Community pharmacy and pharmacist attitudes. *The Pharmaceutical Journal* 1990; 244 (suppl): R7-R10

23. Consumers' Association. Pharmacists: how reliable are they? *Which? Way to Health* 1991; December: 191-194.

24. Goodburn E, Mattosinho S, Mongi P, Waterston T. Management of childhood diarrhoea by pharmacists: is Britain lagging behind the Third World? *British Medical Journal* 1991; 302: 440-443.

25. Smith FJ. Management of childhood diarrhoea. *British Medical Journal* 1991; 302: 788.

26. Mulligan G, Hunt AJ, Herring CN. Responding to ocular symptoms – a survey of community pharmacists. *The Pharmaceutical Journal* 1991; 247 (suppl): R15.

27. Smith FJ. A study of the advisory and health promotion activity of community pharmacists: Cough Symptoms. *Health Education Journal* 1992; 51: 68-71.

28. Anderson CW, Alexander AM. Response to dysmenorrhoea: An assessment of knowledge and skills. *The Pharmaceutical Journal* 1992; 249 (suppl): R2.

29. Alexander AM. The Agent Provocateur study as a research tool. *The Pharmaceutical Journal* 1991; 247: 154-155.

30. Smith FJ, Salkind MR, Jolly BC. Community Pharmacy: a method of assessing quality of care. *Social Science and Medicine* 1990; 31: 603-607.

31. Office of Population Censuses and Surveys. *Mortality Statistics 1990.* London: HMSO; 1991.

32. Townsend P, Davidson N. eds. *The Black Report.* London: Penguin Books; 1982.

33. Whitehead M. *The Health Divide.* London: Penguin Books; 1988.

34. Thorogood M, Coulter A, Muir J, Mant D. Uptake of health checks in General Practice: Does the inverse care law hold true? Proceedings of the 36th Annual Scientific Meeting of the Society for Social Medicine 1992; p25 (unpublished).

35. Nuffield Committee of Inquiry into Pharmacy. *Pharmacy: A report to the Nuffield Foundation.* London: The Nuffield Foundation; 1986.

36. Government White Paper. *Promoting Better Health: The Government's Programme for improving Primary Health Care.* London: HMSO (Cmd 249); 1987.

37. Beattie A. Knowledge and Control in health promotion: a test case for social policy and social theory. In: Gabe J, Calnan N, Bury M. eds. *The Sociology of the Health Service.* London: Routledge; 1991.

38. Szasz TS, Hollender MH. A contribution to the philosophy of medicine: the basic models of the doctor–patient relationship. *Archives of Internal Medicine* 1956; 97: 585-592.

39. Korsch BM, Gozzi EK, Francis V. Gaps in Doctor –Patient communication: Doctor–patient interaction and patient satisfaction. *Pediatrics* 1968; 42: 855-871.

40. Smith FJ. Community Pharmacists and Health Promotion: A study of consultations between pharmacists and clients. *Health Promotion International* 1992; 7: 249-255.

41. Cartwright A, O'Brien M. Social class variations in health care and in general practitioner consultations. In: Stacey M. ed. *The Sociology of the NHS*, Sociological Review Monograph No. 22. Keele: University of Keele; 1976.

42. Bannerman RH, Burton J, Wen-Chieh C. *Traditional Medicine and Health Care Coverage.* Geneva: World Health Organisation; 1983.

43. Fuller JHS, Toon P. *Medicine in a Multicultural Society.* London: Heinemann; 1988.

44. Brent Community Health Council. *Black People and the Health Service.* London: Brent Community Health Council; 1981.

45. Walker IM, Aslam M, Davis SS. Use of a Bradford pharmacy by the Asian and indigenous populations. *The Pharmaceutical Journal* 1980; 225: 703-706.

46. Ronalds C, Vaughan JP, Sprackling P. Asian mothers' use of GP maternal/child welfare services. *Journal of the Royal College of General Practitioners* 1977; 27: 409-416.

47. Aslam M, Healy M. Asiatic medicine. *Update* 1983; 27: 1043-1048.

48. McKinlay TB. Social networks, lay consultation and health seeking behaviour. *Social Forces* 1977; 51: 275-292.

49. Zola I. Pathways to the doctor: from person to patient. *Social Science and Medicine* 1973; 7: 677-689.

50. Hannay DR. *The Symptom Iceberg.* London: Routledge, Kegan and Paul; 1979.
51. Smith FJ. The Community Pharmacist in the Lay – Professional Referral Network. *The Pharmaceutical Journal* 1990; 245 (suppl): R31.
52. Cunningham-Burley S, Maclean U. The role of the chemist in primary health care for children with minor complaints. *Social Science and Medicine* 1987; 24: 371-377.
53. Selya RM. Pharmacies as alternative sources of medical care: the case of Cincinnati. *Social Science and Medicine* 1988; 26: 409-416.
54. Smith FJ. Referral of clients by community pharmacists in primary care consultations. *International Journal of Pharmacy Practice* 1993; 2: 86-89.
55. Smith FJ. Community Pharmacists and Health Visitors: Partnership. *Health Visitor* 1990; 63: 383-384.
56. Smith FJ. Community Liaison: pharmacists and primary health care for children. *Community Outlook* 1993; 3: 39-40.
57. Anonymous. Welsh Pharmaceutical Conference: President calls for private consultation points in all pharmacies. *The Pharmaceutical Journal* 1983; 231: 442.
58. Anonymous. A need for privacy. *The Pharmaceutical Journal* 1992; 249: 701.
59. Dhalla M. Areas for consultations. *The Pharmaceutical Journal* 1992; 249: 715-720.
60. Smith FJ, Salkind MR. Counselling Areas in Community Pharmacies: Views of Pharmacists and Clients. *The Pharmaceutical Journal* 1988; 241: R7.
61. Anonymous. Consultation areas wanted by pharmacists' customers: Grampian Local Health Council survey. *The Pharmaceutical Journal* 1993; 250: 491.
62. Hargie O, Morrow N, Woodman C. Consumer perceptions of and attitudes to community pharmacy services. *The Pharmaceutical Journal* 1992; 249: 688-691.

CHAPTER EIGHT

DO PHARMACY CUSTOMERS REMEMBER THE INFORMATION GIVEN TO THEM BY THE COMMUNITY PHARMACIST?

Alison Blenkinsopp, Elizabeth Robinson and Rhona Panton

INTRODUCTION

During the 1980s there was an increasing awareness within the pharmacy profession of the need for community pharmacists to develop interpersonal skills to enable better communication with their customers. At that time two of the authors Alison Blenkinsopp (AB) and Rhona Panton (RP) were providing continuing education programmes for community and hospital pharmacists in the West Midlands. Interactive training sessions on interpersonal skills were offered based on the work of Morrow and Hargie[1]. In our discussions about methods of evaluating the training we wondered about the feasibility of a before/after comparison of pharmacists' performance. That led us to seek the advice of a psychologist Elizabeth Robinson (ER). Together we decided that the initial research idea would require a larger-scale study than we were able to undertake. However our discussions culminated in a proposal to investigate the extent to which pharmacy customers were able to recall the information and advice given to them. Anecdotal claims have been made that in the relatively informal setting of the pharmacy more questions are likely to be asked of the pharmacist, and more information recalled subsequently, than in the general practitioner surgery environment.

ER's previous research with general medical practitioners[2,3,4] on doctor-patient communication included measurement of patient recall following a consultation with the general practitioner. Robinson and Whitfield[2,3] suggested various reasons why patients might leave a consultation with their general practitioner without asking clarifying questions. Patients may fully understand what they have been told. On the other hand they may have processed information and instructions too superficially to be aware of any problems. The community pharmacist is the last contact in the treatment sequence and the pharmacist has the opportunity to:

i.   support, clarify and supplement the information already given by the general practitioner; through repetition of information and supplementary discussion
ii.   increase understanding and awareness
iii. potentially counteract any effects of time constraints and social distance in the general practitioner consultation.

OBJECTIVES OF THE RESEARCH

Our objectives were to:

i   determine the topics, incidence and circumstances of pharmacist–customer communication
ii.   determine any relationship between the extent to which the customer took an active part in the conversation and their subsequent level of recall
iii. test the effect of the environment in which information is given (medicines counter, counselling area) on customer recall
iv.   identify the extent to which customers welcomed information given by the pharmacist
v.   explore the effectiveness of pharmacists' information–giving to customers, using customer recall as a measure.

METHODS

Selection of Methodology

We decided that in order to analyse the content of pharmacists' discussions with their customers we would need to make recordings in the pharmacy using either audio or video tape. While audio recording had been conducted in community pharmacy[5] we could find no instances of the use of video recording. The potential ethical problems arising from the use of video and its visual identification of individuals (see Ethical considerations, below) led us to adopt audio recording and we obtained information about the equipment used in previous studies.[5]

To minimise disruption to the normal working procedures within the pharmacy, discussions between pharmacist and customer were tape recorded using a remote microphone usually worn by the pharmacist, or, when more than one pharmacist was on duty, placed in a strategic position on the counter. The tape recorder was located in the dispensary and was not visible to customers.

Ethical Considerations

Clearly there are questions of confidentiality involved in conducting research where recordings of pharmacist–customer discussions are made. Any consideration of research ethics requires subjects' rights to be taken into account and it could be argued that consent should be obtained from individuals before recordings were made. While the pharmacists who took part in our studies were aware of the purpose and content of the research there remained a need to inform customers that the research was being carried out. We rejected the concept of requesting individual consent on the grounds that it would disrupt the pharmacy's normal work flow and change fundamentally the nature of the pharmacist–customer interaction. Nevertheless we accepted that customers must be able to decline to participate. In order to do this the pharmacy displayed a prominent notice while recordings were being made. The purpose of the notice was to tell customers about the research, assure them of anonymity and confidentiality and suggest that they should tell the pharmacist if they did not wish to take part. The pharmacist would then switch off the microphone (in the event, no customer notified the pharmacist that they did not want to take part)*

Negotiation of Access

For the initial pilot study AB and RP wrote to five community pharmacists in the West Midlands and visited them to tell the pharmacists about the research and seek their participation and two agreed to take part. Four observation sessions, each of three hours were carried out in two pharmacies. Information was recorded manually including the incidence and purpose of transactions; topics discussed by customers, pharmacists and assistants; whether customers had contact with pharmacists or assistants; whether discussion was initiated by pharmacists, assistants or customers. Subsequently a further four, three-hour sessions were conducted in which manual recording was supplemented by audio tape recording.

For the main studies the researcher wrote to eleven community pharmacists in the West Midlands and Worcestershire and invited them to take part in a research project concerned with advice-giving in community pharmacies. Nine declined to participate, citing concerns about possible damage to relationships with customers and about customers' privacy. Two agreed and subsequently took part in the research.

---

* The wording of the notice was: "This pharmacy has been selected to take part in a study of information given to and needed by customers in pharmacies. This morning/afternoon conversations between the pharmacist and customers will be tape-recorded. If you would prefer not to take part please tell the pharmacist. The recordings will be used with discretion and individual customers will not be named.

Procedure

Transactions relating to prescription and "over-the-counter" medicines were recorded in two sessions, each of three hours duration, with the researcher present as observer. Generally recordings were made between 9.00 am and 12.00 noon or 3.30 pm and 6.30 pm, when pharmacists reported that their pharmacies were most likely to be busy. Details of events, such as links for discontinuous transactions were noted by the researcher to facilitate transcription. The tapes were then transcribed, and the transcripts coded and analysed.

Customer recall was tested by telephone interview the day after the pharmacy visit. After each recorded transaction in which the pharmacist gave advice, instructions or information, the customer was approached by the researcher who invited him/her to take part in a telephone interview the next day. Interviews were recorded with the customer's permission, using a Geemark automatic telecorder then transcribed and analysed. Interviewees were asked "I'm interested in how much you can remember of what the pharmacist said to you yesterday. What can you remember?" Probes were used – "Is there anything else you can remember?", "So that's everything you can remember of what s/he said?" Customers were also asked whether they had found out everything they needed to know about the medicine and if not, had they realised this while in the pharmacy or subsequently. They were also asked about how often they took medicines, their age and current or most recent occupation. Finally, their attitude to the information given by the pharmacist was probed and they were asked whether they welcomed information-giving by the pharmacist.

Coding and Analysis of Data

Transactions were classified as "basic" when there was the minimum of spoken communication, for example, size/brand information for over-the-counter sales and these were discarded from the analyses. Transactions in which more than basic spoken information was exchanged were classified as "extended" when they were customer or pharmacist initiated, and involved further communication through questioning or the introduction of information. The latter comprised 50% of all transactions and it was these we focused on in our analyses. These transactions were classified according to whether the interaction related to a prescription or to self-medication.

Customers were classified as either "active" or "passive" depending on the extent to which they introduced topics into the conversation. Customers were further categorised according to the number of medicines discussed. Simple frequency counts of communication episodes do not reflect the quality and quantity of extended communication within each episode. In our studies some transactions consisted of one phrase, for example, "Take one four times a day", while others lasted for ten to fifteen minutes. Information items given by the pharmacist were coded as "units". An information "unit" was defined as a phrase which, standing alone, could be considered meaningful (and so could be remembered). Each information unit was coded as "essential" or "secondary" and essential information was sub-categorised as "procedural" and "explanatory". Examples of procedural items included how much medicine should be taken or used, how, when and how often it should be taken.

Explanatory items included information about the purpose and expected effect of the medicine; food, drink and other activities to be avoided while taking it; whether it could be taken in combination with other medicines; possible side effects. Content analysis data from the pilot study produced the following categories which were used to code data in the later studies: symptom-related; medication-related; and general topics.

Following each telephone interview the information recalled by the customer was compared with that given by the pharmacist and the level of accuracy of recall was noted. Information items given to and correctly recalled by each customer were coded and counted. Misreported or omitted items were treated as forgotten. Given the limitations on space, we will outline the basis of each study and consider here the key findings from the research and their implications. More detailed results are available in the published research findings[6] and a research thesis.[7]

FINDINGS

There were more prescription customers than self-medication and more of the former were passive, more of the latter, active. Generally recall was low, with only about one-third of the information given being remembered. Customers who took an active part in discussion with pharmacists were likely to receive more information and within this, more items classified as essential. Although customers who took an active part in discussion with pharmacists were likely to receive more information than passive customers, our findings showed that they did not recall significantly more. Much information, including essential items, was forgotten. A comparison between prescription and self-medication customers who took an active part in discussion found no significant differences in the amounts of information received.

The pharmacists in our studies were more likely to initiate extended communication relating to prescribed medicines, while their customers were more likely to initiate extended communication on self-medication. The researcher commented on the time pressures to which the pharmacist was subject, with customers often appearing impatient to receive their prescribed medicines. She postulated that pharmacists might limit extended communication in order not to keep customers waiting too long.

Study One

This study focused on customer participation level and subsequent recall, exploring the influence of experience of medicine use and the number of medicines discussed. Experience was defined by customers' reported frequency of medicine use. Eleven recording and observation sessions, of two hours' duration, were carried out in two pharmacies. It was predicted that customers who were experienced in medicine use would remember more information than those who were not.

Fifty-four customers were approached for interview, of whom forty-six (85%) agreed. Two customers refused outright, others did not have a telephone or said they would be unavailable. Forty-four interviews were successfully completed with adults of average age 41 years (range 19 to 80 years), and thirty-two were female. Based on their occupation 55% were working class, 20% skilled working class, 16% lower middle class and 9% middle class.

There were 28 passive and 16 active customers whose transactions involved prescription medicines in 31 cases, over-the-counter medicines in 11 cases and both in 2 cases. The numbers of items given to both passive and active customers were positively related to the numbers recalled. On average, passive customers received significantly less information than active customers, 8.5 and 15.9 items respectively and recalled less, 2.7 and 4.4 items. The findings are summarised in Table 1.

Table 1: Average amounts of information received, remembered and forgotten by passive and active customers (Study 1)

	Passive	Range	Active	Range
	n = 28		n = 16	
Given	8.5	3–19	15.9	6–30
Recalled	2.7	0–8	4.4	1–11
Forgotten	5.8	1–15	11.6	2–20

Overall, more essential than secondary information was recalled, although average quantities given were not significantly different. Thirteen passive and six active customers who reported that they used medicines frequently were classified as "experienced". Although not found to be related directly to recall, experience was found to be related to participation and the amount of information given.

Study Two

This study aimed to further explore the relationship between number of medicines discussed and recall, and the previous use of the medicine being discussed and general experience of medicine use with subsequent recall. It was predicted that customers who had previous experience with the specific medicine being discussed would remember more than those who did not have such experience. Similarly, we expected that those customers who had general experience of medicine use would remember more than those who did not.

The study also aimed to examine the effect of potentially distracting factors which were internal and external to customers. It was hypothesised that customers' recall would be reduced by distracters such as feeling unwell or being in a hurry, either in the pharmacy or at subsequent interview. It was also predicted that customers who had already received the information about the medicine from their general practitioner would remember more than those who had not had the information repeated in this way. Finally, it was predicted that those customers who reported that they welcomed the information given by the pharmacist would remember more than those who reported that they did not welcome the information. Three recording sessions, each of five hours' duration were carried out in one pharmacy where three pharmacists were on duty.

Sixty-four customers were approached for interview of whom fifty agreed to be interviewed (78%). Nine refused and five did not have a telephone. Seven were not available when followed up, and one transaction was inaudible and was excluded. Thus 42 completed transcripts were analysed, with customers' average age 48 years (range 18-85 years). As in study 1, respondents were mainly working class. The findings relating to customers' welcoming or otherwise the information given by the pharmacist are shown on Table 2.

The lowest level of recall in the analysis as a whole was that of the seven customers who reported that they did not welcome the information given by the pharmacist. Of these seven, four failed to recall any of the items, compared with two of the thirty-five reporting that the information was welcomed. The highest

Table 2: Average amounts of information given, remembered and forgotten in relation to customers' reports of whether the information was welcomed (Study 2)

	Information welcomed n = 35	Information not welcomed n = 7	
Given	10.9	7.9	$p > 0.1$
Recalled	4.2	1.1	$p < 0.02$
Forgotten	6.7	6.7	

level of recall was found in passive customers who reported not having previously received information from their general practitioner. Active customers' recall was low where no information had been given by the general practitioner. Not having recent information to build on, the framing of questions and comments by active customers might have required more thought, competing and interfering with processing of incoming information.

The following variables were found to be unrelated to recall of information: customers' reports of general and specific experience with medicine use; attention distracters such as feeling unwell or being in a hurry in the pharmacy or at interview; whether or not the medicine was for the customer's own use; and whether or not the information from the pharmacist was expected.

Study Three

The final study examined the effect of the environment in which information was given. A comparison was made within one pharmacy where information could be given by the same pharmacist in one of two areas: a sales area where prescriptions were handed out and in a separate counselling area. Seven two-hour recording sessions were conducted.

It was predicted that customers who received information in the counselling area would be more likely to take an active part in discussion with the pharmacist and would receive and remember more information. In the counselling area, it was hypothesised, the pharmacist would feel it was appropriate to give more information, to which customers would be more attentive. In a situation with fewer external distractions in the form of the presence of other customers and transactions it was predicted that there would be more efficient processing of information, leading to better recall.

Thirty-two customers were approached for interview in the counselling area and thirty-three in the sales area. In the counselling area group two declined to take part, one did not have a telephone and two were unavailable at follow-up. Thus twenty-seven interviews were completed. For the sales area group four

Table 3: Information received and recalled by passive and active customers in sales and counselling areas (Study 3).

	Sales area		Counselling area	
	Passive n = 12	Active n = 13	Passive n = 15	Active n = 12
Given	8.9	10.3	8.0	10.7
Recalled	3.8	3.6	3.1	3.3

customers declined to take part and two did not have a telephone. Two were unavailable at follow-up and twenty-five interviews were completed.

The proportions of passive and active customers, those aged under and over forty and male or female were not significantly different in the counselling area and sales area groups. The results are summarised in Table 3.

There were no significant differences in the amounts of essential and secondary information received and recalled by customers in the sales and counselling areas; nor in relation to the effect of customers' participation level.

DISCUSSION AND IMPLICATIONS FOR PHARMACY PRACTICE

The key trigger to information-giving by pharmacists appeared to be the apparent responsiveness of their customers. More information items were therefore given to customers who actively participated in the conversation and such customers recalled a greater number of items than did passive customers. However since active customers received more information they also forgot a large number of items and some important items were incorrectly remembered. Average levels of recall were low with few differences between the groups studied even when there were optimum conditions in terms of reduced distractions and increased privacy.

The average customer recalled three or four items of information and items classified as essential were often forgotten. One conclusion which might be drawn from these findings is that pharmacists should limit the number of items offered and restrict these to essential items only. However this would be a simplistic approach, taking account of neither the pharmacist's role as a provider of information nor the desirability of customers taking the responsibility for seeking the information they consider to be most relevant to their needs.

Our expectation that information given in the counselling area would be better retained, proved not to be supported. Although counselling areas provide increased privacy and appear to be welcomed by many pharmacy customers they may not influence recall. Most of the variables which could have been a distraction to customers and prevent effective information processing appeared not to be so.

During transcription of the pharmacy recordings the rapidity with which information was given by pharmacists was noted by the researcher, who also observed this phenomenon during pharmacy visits. This high-speed delivery probably reflects the time pressure perceived by pharmacists in talking with one customer and aware that there are others waiting for prescriptions to be dispensed. Speed of delivery could undoubtedly have presented an overload on customers' capacity to register and process incoming information. Even if the items had been registered and available in memory there might have been insufficient opportunity for efficient organisation, making retrieval from memory more difficult. Operating constraints may prevent pharmacists' tailoring of their information giving to customers' needs.

Ley's work[8] and that of Raynor[9] on the effectiveness of written information about medicines showed that the giving of such information has the potential to increase patients' knowledge and compliance. Although Ley identified shortcomings in the presentation, language and format of examples studied, he concluded that written information could be an effective supplement to oral information. Written information was not routinely offered in any of the pharmacies we studied.

Pharmacists support, clarify, reinforce and supplement information given by general practitioners. They could link written information to oral instructions and advice which could then act as a focus of attention in the pharmacy and an aid to memory afterwards. Pharmacists could actively explain the purpose and value of written information to customers and encourage its use.

The results of our research suggest that if pharmacists are to be more effective as providers of information about medicines and health, ways need to be identified of ensuring that patients remember and understand the information offered. We believe that further consideration now needs to be given to:

i.   Ways of identifying patients who wish to receive information/advice from the pharmacist
ii.   Ways of presenting oral information so that recall is improved
iii.   The effects on recall of supplementing information given orally by written materials
iv.   The influence of speed of delivery of oral information on recall levels, with the aim of identifying optimum conditions for delivery of oral information in the pharmacy setting.

Our work offers pharmacists scope for reflection on the way in which they give information to their customers and the extent to which that information is remembered. In our view, while many questions remain unanswered, some indicators have been identified with which to analyse current practice and facilitate change.

REFERENCES

1. Morrow NC, Hargie ODW. *Communication skills training for professionals – An instructor's handbook*. London: Chapman and Hall; 1989.
2. Robinson EJ, Whitfield M. Improving the efficiency of patients' comprehension monitoring: a way of increasing patients' participation in general practice consultations. *Social Science and Medicine* 1985; 31: 915-919.

3. Robinson EJ, Whitfield M. Participation of patients during general practice consultation. *Psychology and Health* 1987; 1: 123-132.

4. Robinson EJ, Whitfield MJ. Participation of patients during general practice consultations: Comparison between trainees and experienced doctors. *Family Practice* 1987; 4: 5-10.

5. Smith FJ, Salkind MR. Presentation of clinical symptoms to community pharmacists in London. *Journal of Social and Administrative Pharmacy* 1990; 7: 221-224.

6. Wilson M, Robinson EJ, Blenkinsopp A, Panton RS. Customers' recall of information given in community pharmacies. *International Journal of Pharmacy Practice* 1992; 1: 152-157.

7. Wilson M. *Customers' recall of information given by community pharmacists.* MSc thesis: University of Birmingham; 1990.

8. Ley P. Patients' understanding and recall. In: Pendleton D, Hasler J. eds. *Doctor–patient communication.* London: Academic Press; 1983.

9. Raynor DK. *Patient information and its influence on medication compliance.* PhD thesis: University of Bradford; 1991.

CHAPTER NINE

PHARMACIST–PATIENT COMMUNICATION: THE INTERPERSONAL DIMENSIONS OF PRACTICE

Owen Hargie and Norman Morrow

INTRODUCTION

During the last three decades pharmacy practice has become markedly differentiated, with pharmacists seeking careers, not only in the traditional areas of hospital and community practice, but in science, in the pharmaceutical industry, in management, in clinical pharmacy, in business and in research. Change has occurred not only at the global level but also at grass roots level where, for example, particularly in community practice, time-honoured compounding skills have been taken over by technological advances. In addition, the discovery of new drugs, the complexity of therapeutics, the information explosion, the emergence of biopharmaceutics and pharmacokinetics and the growth of health education services, rank among the factors influencing the change from a 'product'-oriented service to a 'patient'-oriented service.

Pharmaceutical education has had to change in response to these new movements. Traditionally the social sciences have not played a very important role in the majority of pharmacy schools. In effect, pharmacy education has majored on the cognitive and technical or manipulative skills required by the profession at the expense of social or communication skills training. At best it has been assumed that training in communication was 'hidden' within the overall curriculum, in that it is indirectly dealt with in the discussion of various topics, and at worst, there has been the belief that intelligent people (such as pharmacy undergraduates) do not need training in communication.

However, there is now a wider appreciation of the role of communication in the delivery of health care particularly in relation to the interpersonal skills of health professionals. The former reliance upon a medical model of care has been replaced by a more patient-centred approach in which the relationship with patients is seen as an important part of treatment.[1] The impetus to improve communication has also been stimulated by a more consumerist attitude on the part of patients who are now much more prepared to question services and indeed treatments.[2] Furthermore, within the U.K. the Patients' Charter[3] has articulated what members of the public are entitled to, by way of health care provision.

As Smith and Bass[4] have pointed out:

> 'Much of health care is communication centred. As a health professional you give directions, offer reassurances, provide consolation, commiserate, interpret, receive information and carry out directions. The more effectively and efficiently you learn to communicate, the more accomplished you become in fulfilling your health service role.'

There is therefore a number of reasons as to why pharmacists need to pay more attention to their relationships with patients. Another factor may be financial, in that research in the U.S.A. has shown that many patients use mail order services to obtain their medicines.[5,6] Associated with this trend has been patients' expressed dissatisfaction with pharmacist communication. This underlines the need for pharmacists to be more than dispensers of medicines, since as Leufkins[7] has pointed out: 'pharmacists who have the will and opportunity to expand their patient oriented services can expect an improvement in their image as health professionals.' It has also been shown that compliance with prescribed medical regimens improves when pharmacists adopt a more active role in the practice setting.[8] Consumer expectation and satisfaction studies have confirmed that there is a clear public demand for pharmacists to devote more time to patient consultations, in which psychosocial, as well as physical, needs are addressed.[9,10]

In their review of the main findings pertaining to patient–practitioner communication, Dickson *et al.*[11] concluded that:

1. Patients tend to be dissatisfied with advice and information received.
2. There is poor compliance with advice given.
3. Patient satisfaction and compliance are related.
4. There is often failure among patients to remember or understand what they have been told.
5. Patient understanding and recall can be improved through better instructional technique, in that:
   - patients remember best the first instructions presented;
   - emphasised instructions are better recalled;
   - repetition of instruction enhances recall;
   - the fewer the instructions given, the greater proportion of information remembered; and,

- simplification of information enhances recall.
6. Practitioners often ignore or fail to fully attend to the psychosocial needs of patients, which in turn leads to alienation from, and dissatisfaction with, medical care.

A final impetus for greater involvement with patients is that some pharmacists have faced legal action due to a failure to counsel patients on prescription drug therapy. Indeed at least ten U.S.A. States have introduced mandatory patient counselling requirements[12] and within the U.K. Scotland is now the first country to have introduced patient counselling as a formal requirement for a community pharmacy practice allowance. In the past the doctor was seen as prescriber and the pharmacist as dispenser of medications. However, recent changes in standards of practice and expectations concerning the pharmacist's role as counsellor may carry with them professional legal responsibilities.

While there is growing consensus of the need for greater communication between pharmacist and patient, few attempts have been made to define what constitutes effective communication within the pharmacy context. The first step in this process is an understanding of what is meant by the term "communication". In social science terminology communication is the scientific study of the production, processing and effects of those systems used by humans to send and receive messages.[13]

Kitching[14], for example, defined communication as the,

'complex interaction process involving the encoding and transmission of a message with a meaning attached to it by some channel from one person to another.........the recipient of a message indicates, by verbal or nonverbal feedback, whether the message has been received, decoded and understood. The feedback allows the original sender to respond in turn and adjust subsequent input (such that) the process involves understanding, meaning and responsiveness'.

In essence, therefore, communication is the ability of the individual to interact effectively with others. The pharmacist needs to be aware of the totality of the detail being provided, to what is said, how it is said and what else is happening while it is being said, in order for effective communication to occur. This raises the question as to whether competence in communication can be achieved and adequately assessed. It is not surprising that this issue has generated considerable opinion given that: 'Competence is an issue both perennial and fundamental to the study of communication'.[15]

In definitions of interpersonal competence two core features tend to be predominant, namely knowledge and skill. The following are typical of such definitions:

'..competence has two dimensions – knowledge and skills. *Knowledge* includes our awareness and understanding of the numerous variables which affect human relationships. *Skills* involve the ability to pragmatically apply, consciously or even unconsciously, our knowledge.'[16]

'Communication competence focuses on the individual's ability and skill, which necessarily includes both knowledge of the social communication rules and the wherewithal to perform in an appropriate manner.' [17]

Competent communication is therefore both culturally and circumstantially determined, such that what constitutes competent social behaviour within one context may be unacceptable in another. In the same way, assessment of the competence of a particular interaction must consider the opinion or world view of the "other". McCroskey[18] summarised communication competence as requiring that the individual has a repertoire of communication skills, has a predisposition towards communicating with others and finally, has the opportunity to communicate competently.

Given these constituents of competent communication, it is evident that a core defining feature of competence is skill to perform the task effectively. However, the definition of interpersonal communication as skill has been the focus of considerable debate with a wide variety of alternative definitions being proffered in the literature. Following a comprehensive review of these definitions and a subsequent analysis of the nature of skill, Hargie[19] defined interpersonal skill as goal-directed, inter-related, contextually appropriate social behaviours which can be learned and which are under the control of the individual. It is useful to consider briefly the six components of skilled performance within this definition and examine their relevance to pharmacy.

1. Goal-directed. Skilled behaviour is purposeful and intentional and is carried out in order to achieve goals. These goals may not always be pursued at a conscious level and indeed one feature of all skilled performance is that goals are subconscious. The skilled car driver is not consciously aware of goals when driving and does not have to consciously think 'I must depress the clutch before I change gear'. Likewise the skilled pharmacist does not have to consciously think 'I want to find out if the patient has understood therefore I must ask a relevant question'.

2. Inter-related. Social skill involves elements of verbal and nonverbal communication which are closely synchronized in order to bring about a desired consequence. For example, the pharmacist's 'guggles' (uh hu, hm hm), headnods and eye contact should be co-ordinated in such a way as to encourage patients to continue talking, thereby providing important additional information about their situation.

3. Appropriate. To be skilled, social behaviour must be appropriate to the situation. A simple example of this is that the pharmacist may wear a swimming costume on the beach but would not do so at work!

4. Behaviours. This is really the essence of skill. We judge whether people are socially skilled or not based upon how they actually behave.

5. Learned. For the most part, behaviours displayed in the social context are learned by a process of modelling or imitating the performance of significant others. Thus a pre-registration pharmacist is likely to observe and copy the styles, strategies and behaviour of experienced practitioners working in the same environment. Given that skills are learned, it is therefore important to identify effective pharmacist performance and teach the relevant skills to pharmacy trainees.

6. Control. Skilful communication demands that individuals have control over their behaviour and learn not just what the appropriate behaviours are but also how and when to use them. Thus an important dimension of skill relates to the timing of certain aspects of performance. For example, the pharmacist who will not be pressurised into supplying an antibiotic without a prescription may allow considerable gaps in the flow of conversation in order to convey assertiveness.

Having identified the defining features of skilled communication, it is important to relate these directly to the practice context and identify what skills constitute effective pharmacist performance.

METHODS FOR IDENTIFYING COMMUNICATION SKILLS

It is now widely accepted that the quality of practitioner–patient communication is fundamental to effective health care.[20] The question then arises as to exactly what constitutes successful interpersonal communication? What distinguishes good performance from poor performance? How can skilled performance be recognised and analysed so that training programmes can be instituted to develop interpersonal competence? What are the elements of the interpersonal process which when integrated form a co-ordinated whole, and result in the goals of each party being achieved? What are the interpersonal skills required by pharmacists and what are the main skill deficits within this profession? Are there specific situations in pharmacy practice which require specialised interpersonal skills?

One system which has been of growing interest in the analysis and identification of core communication issues across a range of professional contexts is the Communication Audit. This is a method which produces a comprehensive analysis of communication structure, flow and practice.[21] The best known audit system is that developed by Goldhaber and Rogers[22] for the International Communication Association. The audit system enables the researcher to: describe actual patterns of communication behaviours; determine the amount of information underload or overload associated with the major topics, sources and channels of communication; evaluate the quality of information communicated from and/or to these sources and the quality of information relationships; identify the operational communication networks and determine potential bottlenecks and gatekeepers of information; identify categories of recurring positive and negative communication episodes; and identify how and in what ways communication processes and procedures can be improved.

Communication audits have proved to be extremely beneficial in charting the actual patterns of communication which occur in any particular context and also in allowing all of the participants to express their views concerning how these could best be improved.[23] It is therefore a method of gaining information in order to solve communication problems and create more efficient and effective ways of communicating. This information can be gathered in a variety of ways. For example, questionnaires can be administered to all participants asking them to evaluate current communication practices and to identify areas of strengths and weaknesses and suggest how improvements could be effected. Similar information can, of course, be obtained from interviews with participants. Other methods for collecting information include actual observation, recording and analysis of interpersonal encounters; diary analysis to ascertain whom individuals have interacted with and how often over a given period of time; and self-recording of interactions by participants on paper following each interactive episode.

Three main styles of approach have been proposed for the purpose of skill identification during interpersonal communication, namely the analytical, the intuitive and the empirical and these can be employed to identify the core skills central to effective practice in any professional context.[24] The analytical method is, in essence, an armchair theoretical approach to social skill identification. It requires no observation or measurement, but is the result of deductive processes based upon delineating the hypothesised purposes of interactive episodes in particular situations and deducing from these the skilled actions deemed essential for effective performance. Thus, it may be considered that some of the objectives in pharmacy practice are to diagnose patient problems, provide information on medication, and encourage compliance with therapy. Following on from this it could then be postulated that the skill concepts of questioning, explaining and influencing will be important elements for the pharmacist to master.

By contrast, the intuitive approach relies upon the intuitions of experienced practitioners to produce a list of appropriate skills for effective performance. It is experiential in nature and relies upon a reflective style of analysis, whereby the experienced professional is encouraged to make comments such as: 'When

I was in that situation I found it was useful to....' It is, therefore, inductive in that as experiences are collated, shared and discussed with other professionals, it is possible to build up a picture of what are generic key skills, and also which situations demand special skills.

The empirical approach is distinct from the former two, as it involves the systematic observation, recording and categorisation of interactions to identify core skills. In other words, this represents the application of the traditional scientific method to the study of interpersonal encounters through the use of behaviour analysis of professional encounters. Within this approach there are two main methodologies which can be employed, namely task analysis and constitutive ethnography. The former involves shadowing someone as they work and noting exactly what tasks are performed. It suffers from the major disadvantage that, while it identifies the functional elements of professional practice, it does not give any indication of the level of skill with which the practitioner performs them, nor does it provide information concerning what constitutes effective practice.

Constitutive ethnography, on the other hand, facilitates the identification and analysis of effective interpersonal communication. This approach, which is part of what is referred to as the "consultative" research paradigm,[25] involves capturing a range of interactive events on video and subsequently subjecting these to intensive peer analysis and evaluation. Thus, the ethnographer is concerned to document at a more micro level the interactional behaviour of participants. It is therefore possible to delineate in detail all of the behaviours deemed essential for effective communication. It is also possible to begin to identify useful strategies for patient consultations which make the interaction more effective and more satisfying for the participants. Moreover, the importance of the nonverbal elements of behaviour can be identified and specific cues which moderate, control and facilitate interactions can be elicited, thereby giving direction to those elements of skilled performance which need to be developed or trained. Overall then, constitutive ethnography involves analysing interpersonal behaviour in order to chart those skills and strategies which go to producing skilled performance at the pharmacist–patient interface.

In relation to the informational role of the pharmacist, Berardo *et al.*[26] identified four main categories of information provided in the course of patient consultation. These were concerned with information about how to take the medication, side effects, dosage and number of doses per day. In addition, they reported that the workload of the pharmacy did not affect the number of dispensing episodes that included consultations with patients. Wilson *et al.*[27] also carried out empirical research in community pharmacies, in which they employed a combination of audio-recording, direct observation and interviews to evaluate patient understanding and recall of instructions and advice given. However, their findings related solely to the imparting of information and did not indicate the nature of the specific communication skills used by participating pharmacists in the course of such interactions.

In another such investigation, audio-recordings were made of over 700 pharmacist–patient interactions in community pharmacies in the London area. It was found that the average duration of consultations was 2.5 minutes.[28] However, in a subset of these consultations dealing specifically with coughs, the contact time fell to 1.6 minutes with pharmacists asking a mean number of 3 questions, and giving an average of 4.4 items of information or advice, per consultation.[29] Furthermore, it has been shown that the amount of time pharmacists spend speaking to patients about medicines is on average 3.5 minutes per hour.[30]

Thus, the main emphasis of most studies has been upon either product information or the volume and throughput of "consumers", with a paucity of research into the skilled nature of communication in pharmacy practice. However, two main methods of enquiry have been implemented to address the latter, both of which have used pharmacists as a core source of expert knowledge for their data analysis, thereby allowing an "inside" view of practice. Firstly, investigations have been undertaken of the accounts of pharmacists regarding their management of core situations and difficulties encountered in the workplace. In these studies pharmacists were requested to reflect back upon the skills and strategies they employed in specific contexts of practice. Secondly, more "invasive" research has been carried out, whereby pharmacists have been required to analyse actual video-recordings of their own consultations with patients and delineate effective skills employed.

The investigation by Morrow and Hargie[31] of critical incidents in the context of pharmacy practice represented an initial attempt to ascertain the pertinent issues of interpersonal communication as perceived by practising pharmacists. Their data, derived from the views of pharmacists working in hospital, community and administrative practice, indicated that pharmacists felt that communication could be hampered because of difficulties experienced in the course of interacting with "problem patients". The problem patients identified included those suffering from drug addiction, depression, disability and terminal illness. The types of communication difficulties presented by these problem patients were classified in terms of difficulties associated with the gathering and giving of information, evaluative difficulties (e.g. the assessment of patient needs and understanding), embarrassing personal problems, dealing with emotional issues and miscellaneous difficulties, which included the resolution of ethical, legal and financial conflicts and time constraints.

In another study using similar methodology, the same authors investigated the counselling dimension of practice.[32] Pharmacists identified and scored those situations where counselling was most frequently indicated and the difficulties encountered in such situations. As can be seen from Tables 1 and 2, the situation

TABLE 1: Rank order of situations where counselling is indicated (adapted from reference 31).

1	Confusion over medication
2	Medication problems in the elderly
3	Anxiety over treatment
4	Medication counselling prior to patient discharge
5	Dissatisfaction with treatment
6	Diabetic patients
7	Patients with cardiovascular disease
8	Dealing with adverse drug reactions
9	Patients using inhalers
10	Cancer patients
11	Terminally ill patients
12	Drug therapy in pregnancy
13	Medication history taking
14	Patients on warfarin therapy
15	Mother/baby problems
16	Patients on steroid therapy
17	Patients using stoma appliances
18	Patients on MAOIs
19	Anxiety over disease prognosis
20	Worried patients
21	Smoking

which was regarded as being most prevalent was that of dealing with confusion over medication, with the second being that of medication problems in the elderly. The two most frequently mentioned counselling difficulties were having sufficient time to deal with patients and ensuring patient understanding.

Using the constitutive ethnography approach to skill identification, Hargie *et al.*[13] videotaped 350 real pharmacist–patient consultations in 15 community pharmacies. These were then subjected to a detailed peer review procedure aimed at identifying the core skills inherent in effective interactions. This resulted in a comprehensive inventory of 45 key behaviours which were categorised into 11 main skill areas (Table 3). The range of skills and sub-skills charted in this research is of particular importance since it is the first

TABLE 2: Rank order of reported counselling difficulties
(adapted from reference 31).

1	Having sufficient time
2	Ensuring patient understanding
3	Dealing with patients' preconceived ideas
4	Overcoming patients' communicative disabilities
5	Lack of liaison with other carers
6	Getting patients to accept responsibility for their own health
7	Deciding depth of involvement
8	Knowing what is the appropriate thing to say
9	Lack of background knowledge of the patient's situation
10	Avoiding causing patient harm
11	Providing privacy
12	Dealing with patients' worries
13	Lack of knowledge to do adequate counselling
14	Fear of impinging on another professional's domain
15	Exploring the situation
16	Giving reassurance
17	Helping the patient to see an appropriate course of action
18	Dealing with an emotional problem
19	Providing empathy
20	Giving support

comprehensive, empirically validated, list of communication competencies. Several notable features were evident from this study.

Firstly, in a number of instances, the same behaviour was categorised by pharmacists under more than one skill area. This underlines the integrative nature of interpersonal performance in that one particular behaviour may help to achieve several goals. Secondly, some behaviours were described by virtue of their verbal content (e.g. questions on symptoms, previous action taken, other medication used), while others were described in communication process terms (e.g. reinforcing, politeness, use of humour). Thus it may be argued that different behaviours were seen either in communication "content" terms or in communication "construction" terms, i.e. the *what* of communication and the *how*. That some categories were sub-divided predominantly into one of either

TABLE 3: Communication skills and sub-skills identified by pharmacists
(adapted from reference 13).

1.	**Questioning**
a	Re: patient details, name, age etc
b	Re: symptoms, previous action taken, cause of health problem, duration, lifestyle, previous action of other health professionals
c	Checking out/exploring situation
d	Showing interest
e	Re: other medication being taken
2.	**Listening**
a	Showing sympathy/empathy
b	Encouraging patient to provide information
c	Showing interest (beyond the problem)
3.	**Assertiveness**
a	Enhancing credibility by referring to view of other health professionals
b	Pharmacist politely standing ground
4.	**Explaining**
a	Reasoned instructions
b	Directing
c	Informing
d	Explaining for reassurance
e	Repetition
f	Reinforcing/emphasising
5.	**Nonverbal communication**
a	Tone of voice
b	Standing still
c	Eye contact
d	Proximity
e	Positioning
f	Smiling and/or nodding head
g	Using hand gestures
h	Touch
i	Illustration/demonstration/display
j	Pharmacist examining patient

6.   Building Rapport

a   Showing genuine concern

b   Showing pleasure/happiness

c   Greeting by name

d   Being helpful

e   Accommodating patient's needs

f   Politeness in manner

g   Use of humour

h   Being available/accessible

i   Engaging

j   Offering reassurance

k   Preserving confidentiality

l   Showing warmth

m   Showing patient interest

7.   Opening

a   Greeting, general

b   Greeting by name

c   Identifying patient by name (script check)

8.   Closing

a   Thanking patient

b   Initiating ending of interaction

c   Polite closing

9.   Suggesting/Advising

10.   Disclosing personal information

11.   Persuading

of these two dimensions was clear. For example, questioning was viewed as a content based skill, whereas explaining was much more a construction based skill.

Thirdly, some skills were perceived as being more complex than others, so that, for example, building rapport had by far the largest number of behavioural sub-categories. It may therefore be postulated that pharmacists regard the relationship element of practice as particularly powerful, such that many strategies are required to initiate, maintain and enhance relationships. Community pharmacy is somewhat unique in that it operates as a helping profession within the realities of business practice. Thus there are two motivations for maintaining patient rapport; one the demonstration of a caring practitioner, and second, the creation and preservation of patient loyalty to achieve business success.

Fourthly, an examination of the levels of skill usage suggested that as frequency of positive skill use increased so did ratings of communication effectiveness. In addition, the results indicated that non-prescription related consultations demanded an extended skill usage. Indeed the skill of suggesting/advising was evident only in these consultations. It may be that part of the reason for these differences is related to the fact that in prescription related instances, the patient has had a consultation with a doctor and therefore comes to the pharmacy better informed. In the other case the patient has taken the initiative to approach the pharmacist and therefore, with patients negotiating their own needs, the pharmacist may have to employ a wider repertoire of skills. It may be argued that in the prescription situation the doctor has given the advice/suggestion in the form of a written order, such that the pharmacist is not centrally involved. In the non-prescription situation however, the pharmacist is playing a role equivalent to the doctor.

Fifthly, based on a frequency of use pattern, *building rapport, explaining* and *questioning* emerged as the core skills adjudged to be central to pharmacy practice. Furthermore, the identification of the skill of *suggesting/advising* is worthy of note, since this is a dimension of communication which has not received any real attention in the health communication literature, and may indeed be a particular feature of community pharmacy practice.

Finally, an extension of this research involved a micro analysis of the questions used in the consultations of five of the participating pharmacists.[33] The results indicated that 98% of all questions asked by pharmacists were closed in nature, over two thirds of which simply required a 'Yes' or 'No' answer. Twenty four percent were phrased in a leading fashion. Only 2% were concerned with the psychosocial aspects of practice with the vast majority focusing purely upon clinical matters. This pattern of questions suggests a particular interviewing style in which the pharmacist controls and directs the consultation. Closed and leading questions restrict the scope of responses and assume prior knowledge on the part of the questioner, such that the information gathered may be incomplete or inaccurate, potentially resulting in compromised action. For this reason pharmacists need to develop effective interviewing techniques which will be *objective* in the collection of data and *open* to the needs of clients.

FUTURE IMPLICATIONS

Research into the identification of the core communication skills used by pharmacists in their professional encounters with patients has provided an important focus for training and further research. In relation to the former there are three main reasons why pharmacist training should include a strong communication component. Firstly, the interpersonal nature of the profession demands those skills which will lead to improved communicative performance. Secondly, and linked to this, is the ability to allow patients to negotiate their own needs and produce satisfaction. Thirdly, without a knowledge of the nature of interpersonal skill, pharmacists will not be able to evaluate their own or others' communicative behaviour and performance.

Some ten years ago the Pharmaceutical Society of Great Britain Working Party report on pharmaceutical education and training[34] stressed the importance of developing the interpersonal skills of students and graduates, pointing out that without such skills pharmacists would not have received an adequate preparation for practice. This report asserted that without effective communication skills pharmacists would: 'not have the basis for the provision of the full range of professional services which should be available in community practice'. Indeed, a satisfactory level of communication skills was suggested as a criterion for graduation and professional registration by the report of this Working Party, which stated: '...it will be even more important in the future for students to be able to communicate satisfactorily with the public and with members of other health professions. Otherwise they should not expect to graduate and register.'

This was supported in the report of the Nuffield Committee of Inquiry into Pharmacy[35] which stressed the importance of communication to effective practice and clearly identified 'pharmacy's neglect of its own social context, and social science's neglect of pharmacy'. The report advocated that the pharmacy curriculum should be restructured to include the teaching of behavioural sciences especially in relation to the behaviour of health care professionals and patients. Specific attention was also drawn to the importance and need to develop communication skills training as part of both undergraduate and postgraduate education. The Committee recommended the testing of oral skills at the end of the pre-registration period, which students would have to successfully complete before registration. Furthermore, the Inquiry Committee recommended that 'research into pharmacy practice in co-operation with social and behavioural scientists should be increased'. The importance of these issues was reinforced in the same year by the Government's discussion paper on Primary Health Care[36] which highlighted the need for pharmacists' training to supplement their scientific training with skills relevant to their wider roles, that is, skills in communication, counselling and behavioural science.

Despite these recommendations, it is still possible for pharmacists to graduate and register without having demonstrated communicative competence to a prescribed level. As many medicines will move from Prescription Only Medicines to Pharmacy Medicines, the advisory role of the pharmacist will become more dominant, and the need for advisory skills (both clinical and interpersonal) more prominent. Research has shown a clear public demand for easier access to, and direct contact with, pharmacists as distinct from counter staff, and a desire for the pharmacist to address psychosocial needs.[9] Given the incontrovertible evidence regarding the importance of communication to effective practice, coupled with increased public expectations, it is inevitable that in future pharmacists will be assessed on their professional interpersonal skills. It is therefore vital that communication skills training should become formalised in the undergraduate curriculum with refresher training at post-qualification level.

While recent research has produced valuable information pertaining to pharmacist communication, some of the key research questions which remain to be answered include the following:

1. To what extent do pharmacists recognise and deal with the psychosocial aspects of practice?
2. Precisely how do prescription-related situations differ from non-prescription related interactions in terms of interactive patterns?
3. What situations in pharmacy demand special skills?
4. How is practice to be developed to build rapport with the public?
5. How is practice changing traditionally held pharmacy beliefs?
6. How can communicative competency best be measured prior to qualification?
7. In what ways does the nature of communication change from one branch of pharmacy practice to another?

Thus, more extensive research is needed in order to gain as full a picture as possible of those factors which contribute to success or failure in practice. Presently, pharmacy lags behind other health professions, where such research has already been carried out. It is only by conducting concerted research in this field that future practitioners can be fully equipped to meet real world practice needs.

REFERENCES

1. Stewart M, Roter D, eds. *Communicating with medical patients.* Newbury Park: Sage; 1989.
2. Armstrong D. What do patients want? *British Medical Journal* 1991; 303: 261-262.
3. Department of Health. *The Patients' Charter.* London: HMSO; 1991.
4. Smith V, Bass T. *Communication for the health care team.* London: Harper and Row; 1982.
5. Enriquez N. Post-script – don't forget to listen. *Hospital Pharmacy* 1986; 21: 35.

6. Dickinson J. Patient relations: the core of your practice. *U.S. Pharmacist* 1987; 12: 28-30.
7. Leufkins HGM. Patient counselling and the public image of the pharmacist. *Pharmaceutisch Weekblad* 1986; 121: 514-519.
8. Berger B, Felkey B. A conceptual framework for focusing the teaching of communication skills and compliance-gaining strategies. *American Journal of Pharmaceutical Education* 1989; 53: 259-265.
9. Hargie ODW, Morrow NC, Woodman C. Consumer perceptions of and attitudes to community pharmacy services. *The Pharmaceutical Journal* 1992; 249: 688-691.
10. Hargie ODW, Morrow NC, Woodman C. Consumer perceptions of and attitudes to the advice-giving role of community pharmacists. *The Pharmaceutical Journal* 1993; 251: 25-27.
11. Dickson DA, Hargie ODW, Morrow NC. *Communication skills training for health professionals: an instructor's handbook.* London: Chapman and Hall; 1989.
12. Simonsmeier LM. Topic update on: legal issues surrounding the pharmacist's duty to counsel patients, employment law and mail order pharmacy. *American Journal of Pharmaceutical Education* 1989; 53: 73-77.
13. Hargie ODW, Morrow NC, Woodman C. *Looking into community pharmacy: identifying effective communication skills in pharmacist–patient consultations.* Jordanstown: University of Ulster; 1993.
14. Kitching J. Communication and the community pharmacist. *The Pharmaceutical Journal* 1986; 237: 449-452.
15. Spitzberg B, Cupach W. *Interpersonal communication competence.* Beverly Hills: Sage; 1984.
16. Konsky C, Murdock J. Interpersonal communication. In: Cragan F, Wright D, eds. *Introduction to speech communication.* Illinois: Waveland Press; 1980.
17. Wiemann J, Backlund P. Current theory and research in communication competence. *Review of Educational Research* 1980; 50: 185-199.
18. McCroskey J. Communication competence: the elusive construct. In: Bostrom R, ed. *Communication: a multidisciplinary approach.* Beverly Hills: Sage; 1984.
19. Hargie O. ed. *A handbook of communication skills.* London: Routledge; 1986.
20. Ley P. *Communicating with patients.* London: Croom Helm; 1988.
21. Emmanuel M. Auditing communication practices. In: Reuss C, DiSilvas R, eds. *Inside organisational communication.* London: Longman; 1985.
22. Goldhaber G, Rogers D. *Auditing organizational communication systems: the International Communication Audit.* Texas: Kendall Hunt; 1979.
23. Downs CW. *Communication audits.* Illinois: Scott/Foresman; 1988.
24. Ellis R, Whittington D. *A guide to social skill training.* London: Croom Helm; 1981.
25. Caves R. Consultative methods for extracting expert knowledge about professional competence. In: Ellis R, ed. *Professional competence and quality assurance in the caring professions.* London: Croom Helm; 1988.
26. Berardo D, Kimberlin C, Barnett CW. Observational research on patient education activities of community pharmacists. *Journal of Social and Administrative Pharmacy* 1989; 6: 21-30.
27. Wilson M, Robinson EJ, Ellis A. Studying communication between community

pharmacists and their customers. *Counselling Psychology Quarterly* 1989; 2: 367-380.

28. Smith F. Community pharmacists and health promotion: a study of consultations between pharmacists and clients. *Health Promotion International* 1992; 7: 249-255.

29. Smith FJ. A study of the advisory and health promotion activity of community pharmacists. *Health Education Journal* 1992; 51: 68-71.

30. Fisher CM, Corrigan OI, Henman MC. A study of community pharmacy practice (1. Pharmacists' work patterns). *Journal of Social and Administrative Pharmacy* 1991; 8: 15-23.

31. Morrow NC, Hargie ODW. An investigation of critical incidents in interpersonal communication in pharmacy practice. *Journal of Social and Administrative Pharmacy* 1987; 4: 112-118.

32. Morrow NC, Hargie ODW. Patient counselling: an investigation of core situations and difficulties in pharmacy practice. *International Journal of Pharmacy Practice* 1992; 1: 202-205.

33. Morrow NC, Hargie ODW, Donnelly H, Woodman C. 'Why do you ask?' A study of questioning behaviour in community pharmacist–client consultations. *International Journal of Pharmacy Practice* 1993; 2: 90-94.

34. Pharmaceutical Society of Great Britain. First report of the working party on pharmaceutical education and training. *The Pharmaceutical Journal* 1984; 232: 495-508.

35. Nuffield Committee of Inquiry into Pharmacy. *Pharmacy: a report to the Nuffield Foundation*. London: The Nuffield Foundation; 1986.

36. Department of Health and Social Security. *Primary health care: an agenda for discussion*. London: HMSO; 1986.

CHAPTER TEN

THE EFFECTS OF PATIENT INFORMATION LEAFLETS ON CLIENTS' UNDERSTANDING OF METHADONE THERAPY

Kay Roberts and Ivor Harrison

INTRODUCTION

During the 1980s the Royal Pharmaceutical Society of Great Britain recognised the need for pharmacists to become more aware of the problems, issues, and treatment options associated with substance misuse. The Society published "Drug Abuse – A guide for pharmacists"[1] and distributed it to every community pharmacy in Britain together with additional information on treatment and support agencies available locally. In a Policy Statement relating to pharmaceutical supplies for drug misusers,[2] issued in 1991 the Society suggested that such services should be provided by pharmacists who understood and knew the problems associated with substance misuse. One group of drug misusers pharmacists will come into contact with are those on methadone maintenance programmes, who have their prescriptions dispensed from community pharmacies.

Methadone is prescribed to opiate drug misusers as substitution therapy. Unlike morphine or heroin (diamorphine) the drug is as effective orally as when given by injection. Tolerance develops readily, but there is little tendency to increase dose or dose rate as oral methadone does not produce the "rush" associated with injected heroin. Methadone has a longer half-life than heroin, so that withdrawal is less intense. During methadone maintenance therapy the drug user is stabilised on a dose sufficient to suppress heroin withdrawal for 12 to 24 hours but which will not produce the euphoria of opiate drugs. Perhaps methadone's main advantage is that it can counter the withdrawal effects of heroin or other opiates in a single daily oral dose.

Philips *et al.*[3] showed that anxiety-related factors are associated with the severity of withdrawal. However, such distress can be greatly reduced by the provision of accurate and reassuring information to methadone users[4]. Discussions with drug misusers confirmed previous observations that many myths surround the use of methadone in the treatment of opiate dependent drug addiction.[5] There appeared to be a need for an information source to this patient group.

Community pharmacists are one of a group of health professionals likely to come in contact with this client group and indeed provision of health advice and health promotion literature is an integral part of community based pharmaceutical services. Such literature may include patient information leaflets (PILs) used to enhance patient understanding, knowledge, and compliance with medication regimens. Hermann *et al.*[6] suggested that the minimum information contained in PILs should include details of administration and storage, how the treatment is expected to help and how to recognise and deal with possible adverse effects of the therapy.

A study of patients undergoing methadone therapy was therefore conducted to investigate the impact of a PIL on this client group's knowledge of their drug therapy. The aims and objectives of this study were to establish the level of understanding of the drug treatment of a sample of clients receiving prescribed methadone from community pharmacies, and subsequently to re-evaluate their understanding following exposure to a suitably designed PIL.

METHODOLOGY

Prior to designing the leaflet, the views of general practitioners who prescribed for drug misusers and drug workers in five treatment centres were considered and their suggestions incorporated. The leaflet was refined subsequent to piloting and additional information on methadone and driving was obtained from the Medical Officer of the Department of Transport. The final version of the five page leaflet contained information under the following headings: What is methadone? How does methadone work? How can the drug help me? For how long should I take methadone? Will methadone alone cure my problem? What happens if I stop taking methadone? What are the difficulties involved in methadone treatment? Methadone and driving, and methadone collection from pharmacies.

A self administered questionnaire was designed to evaluate this leaflet and given to clients waiting to collect their prescribed medication. Thirty nine community pharmacies and two community drug agencies in North West London where Methadone Mixture 1 mg/ml was dispensed were identified and supplied with copies of the questionnaires and the PIL.

Clients presenting a prescription for Methadone Mixture were given a numbered copy of the questionnaire printed on pink paper. A copy on green paper bearing the same serial number was clipped to the prescription. When the drug was handed out, the pharmacist collected the pink questionnaire, provided the client with a PIL and instructed him/her to read it carefully. When returning to collect their next dose (usually the following day) clients were asked to complete the green copy of the questionnaire, which was collected by pharmacists when handing out that day's supply of methadone. This green questionnaire contained additional questions about the acceptability of the leaflet.

Differences in the responses given in the green and pink questionnaires were recorded using the Statistical Package for the Social Sciences (SPSS-PC) and the data analysed using the McNemar Test which is particularly appropriate in "before and after" study designs where each person acts as their own "control". One disadvantage of the McNemar is that it is a test of dichotomous responses. Where three possible answers could be given, i.e. "yes", "no" and "don't know", it was necessary to re-apply the test to different pairs of responses, e.g. yes/no, yes/don't know.*

RESULTS AND DISCUSSION

Three hundred and eighty four pairs of forms were distributed, of which 119 pink, and 110 green were completed, a response rate of 119/384 (31%) and 110/119 (92%) respectively. However, one of the major difficulties with postal surveys is the interpretation of non-response, the main problem being the inability to distinguish between those who refused to reply and those who were not contacted for one of a variety of reasons. There are several possible different methods for calculating the realism of the response rate. In this research because all forms could be variously accounted for, a formula recommended by Owens *et al*[7] was applied:

---

* The McNemar Test

To test the significance of any observed change by this method a fourfold table of frequencies is set up to represent the first and second set of responses from the same individual. The general features of this table are illustrated below, where + and − are used to signify different responses.

		AFTER	
		−	+
BEFORE	+	A	B
	−	C	D

Those cases which show changes between the first and second response appear in cells A and D. Since A+D represents the **TOTAL** number of persons whose responses changed, the expectation under the null hypothesis (Ho) would be that $1/2(A+D)$ cases changed in one direction and $1/2(A+D)$ cases changed in the other. In other words $1/2(A+D)$ is the expected frequency under Ho in both cell A and cell D. In all examples the combined sum of the figures in boxes A, B, C, and D equals the number of cases for which an exact match was possible.

$$\text{Response Rate} = \frac{\text{Number of Completed Questionnaires}}{\text{Number in Sample (not eligible and not reachable)}}$$

This resulted in a pre-test response rate of 119/141, or 84% on the grounds that at least 243 were "not eligible or not reachable" because forms were either reported lost in the post, the pharmacist had failed to comply with the protocol, or forms were not given out because the estimated number of clients no longer attended the pharmacy.

What Sort of Drug is Methadone?

One hundred and fifteen of the 119 respondents had previously taken methadone, indicating that they had previous experience of the drug. However, there was no significant difference in the knowledge between these respondents and the four who answered that they had not previously received methadone. The large majority correctly identified methadone as an opiate (89%) or a "downer" i.e. depressant (2%). Six per cent believed methadone was a stimulant, which may have been based on a knowledge that methadone made them feel better when they were in withdrawal.

Methadone's Effects on Individuals

To establish the advantages of a methadone programme, clients were asked how methadone could help them. Fifty five per cent of respondents reported that it stabilised their habit, 29% that it was long acting, 67% that it prevented withdrawal, and 40% that it was legal. After reading the leaflet, there was a significant change ($p=<0.05$) in the number of respondents who appreciated that methadone stabilised their habit (70%) and was long acting (41%).

Prior to reading the PIL, the majority (68%) of respondents appreciated that methadone alone would not overcome their addiction, with 20% uncertain. This number fell to 15% on reading the PIL. Further, the majority of respondents (89% pre and 90% post reading the leaflet) appreciated that methadone was not easy "to get off". These included the four respondents who claimed not to have taken methadone previously.

The pharmacological effects of oral methadone mixture are not immediate, although they are relatively prolonged. Sixty three per cent of respondents pre, and 74% post PIL, said that they would not immediately expect to "feel well", after receiving a dose of methadone. Asked whether withdrawal occurred "quickly" or "slowly" when methadone ceased to be taken, 43% believed the onset of withdrawal occurred quickly and 56%, slowly. Having read the PIL there was a significant increase ($p=<0.001$) in those believing that methadone withdrawal occurs slowly (70%). It is possible that some respondents had never experienced "true" withdrawal from methadone and equated the time scale of methadone withdrawal with that of heroin. In this respect, the PIL may have helped to dispel such misconceptions.

The use of methadone would not be expected to cause sleeping difficulties. Prior to and after reading the leaflet 32% and 33% respectively believed methadone would disturb their sleep. Sixty four per cent and 65% respectively said it would not cause sleeping difficulties. The responses to this question were equivocal. For instance, one respondent mentioned sleep problems following excessive doses of methadone whilst another only noticed problems when the dose was omitted or low. Without knowing whether or not these clients were taking other drugs in addition to their methadone, it is difficult to establish whether these are genuine differences in response to the methadone. Also, sleep problems may be due to other life factors. Three respondents mentioned that they experienced occasional problems and one indicated experiencing problems at the start of treatment. Two respondents reported difficulty when taking the drug at night and another reported no difficulties when the dose was taken later in the day. One respondent specifically mentioned experiencing nightmares.

The leaflet indicated that dividing the dose of methadone into two doses, morning and evening, would make sleeping easier. There was a significant (p=<0.05) increase in the number of respondents (43% to 63%) who subsequent to reading the leaflet appreciated that taking methadone later in the day would aid sleep.

Prior to reading the PIL the majority (81%) of respondents felt it was "OK" to drive whilst on methadone, although many qualified their answers. Fourteen suggested that it was "OK" depending on a number of factors including dose, tolerance and when the drug was prescribed. Only four were aware that to drive whilst taking methadone was illegal.

Pre and post leaflet responses were significantly different (p=<0.001). Fifty six per cent believed it "OK" and 33% not "OK" to drive. However, several respondents stated that although they now realised it was "not OK", they believed that it might be "OK" if they were stabilised on the drug. One suggested that it was "OK" to drive if the methadone was prescribed. Six suggested it would be "OK if the dose was correct". Ten believed that tolerance should be taken into account when deciding whether or not it was "OK" to drive.

The participants in the study were asked to briefly describe any difficulties they would expect when taking methadone. Seventeen pre-leaflet forms contained no response to this open question. Twenty-one expected no difficulty but ten of these qualified their answer with comments such as "apart from methadone dependence", "only when not taking methadone are there difficulties" and "I stay normal". The remaining 81 replies fell into the categories of adverse effects, such as constipation, weight gain; and socio-legal difficulties such as having to collect the drug daily, problems when a container was broken, and problems with pharmacy opening times. Many respondents cited more than one difficulty. Thirty five respondents were worried about withdrawal. The replies included concern about specific symptoms (such as cramp and 'flu), the fear of withdrawal, or fear of not being prescribed sufficient methadone to prevent withdrawal.

The withdrawal effects of methadone are slow in onset but longer-lasting than those of heroin.[8] Respondents confirmed the relatively slow onset of withdrawal and many believed methadone was much harder to "get off" than heroin. Several mentioned the disappointment that occurs after managing easily the first two or three days of withdrawal. Gossop *et al.*[9] found that many opiate addicts were frightened of withdrawal, and some respondents did express concern about the possibility of reductions in dosage, delays in dispensing the product, or the consequences of broken container, all of which may precipitate withdrawal.

Twelve respondents commented on the difficulties involved in collecting the drug every day. This was a particular problem for those who were trying to maintain employment. Eight respondents mentioned the loss of excitement and "buzz" associated with heroin use and the difficulties of having to adjust to life without it. Other problems included lack of sex-drive, finding somewhere private to take doses when at work, and keeping out of sight of their children, sickness when methadone was first prescribed, a false sense of reality, socialising without others noticing signs of intoxification, occasional cramps and diarrhoea, taste, scratching, itchiness, travel, weight gain and stabilising one "habit" with another. As the majority of respondents had previously received methadone, these responses were based on problems already encountered rather than on those anticipated.

Twenty post-PIL forms contained no comments on difficulties associated with taking methadone. The responses were similar to those which had been received to the pre-leaflet questionnaire.

Use of other medication whilst taking methadone

When asked whether it was "OK" to take other drugs concurrently with methadone, the pre-leaflet responses indicated that they were uncertain of the associated dangers (40% yes, 35% no, 25% don't know). Fourteen respondents suggested it might be "OK" depending on, for example, commitment to the reduction programme. Fourteen respondents also considered it "OK" with certain drugs. Six mentioned cannabis, four opiates, two benzodiazepines, and two, other drugs also prescribed for them. Four clients recognised the dangers of taking substances in addition to methadone. There was a statistically significant change in knowledge between the pre and post leaflet responses ($p= <0.001$) with 26% indicating it was OK and 66% not OK to take other drugs. In addition there was a significant reduction ($p=<0.001$) in "don't know" answers (8%).

Additional comments to both the pre-and post-test questionnaire appeared to confirm clients' used drugs in addition to methadone. Cannabis use, although not mentioned extensively post-leaflet, appeared to be considered normal. The majority of respondents pre (87%) and post (89%) leaflet were aware that tolerance increases when opiates are used in addition to methadone. Fewer than half the respondents appreciated that drinking alcohol whilst taking methadone resulted in them becoming drunk quicker (36% pre and 46% post leaflet). Fifteen pre leaflet respondents claimed not to know the answer because they did not drink alcohol. This was unexpected as a combined alcohol/drug problem has been previously reported.[10]

The McNemar test showed that there was no significant difference change in knowledge, and similarly no significant change in knowledge was found when clients were asked what happened when they took "uppers" (stimulants, e.g. cocaine, amphetamines) or "downers" (depressants, e.g. barbiturates, tranquillisers and benzodiazepines) at the same time as their methadone.

CONCLUSIONS

Methadone users represent a significant client group for pharmacists, requiring appropriate and comprehensive information about the aims and benefits of methadone maintenance therapy. Certainly, some of the prescribing physicians and drug workers lack a clear understanding of many aspects of the regimen and are therefore unable to respond to common queries, e.g. the requirement of those receiving methadone to inform the DVLA.

It was evident from this survey that participating pharmacists provided a valued service and most respondents saw little scope for any extension or improvement except for the provision of information, though some suggested the potential benefit to them of having a private area within the pharmacy where they could talk with the pharmacist.

The aim of the pre leaflet questionnaire was to ascertain the knowledge, attitudes and beliefs of a group of drug users receiving methadone as part of their treatment. The majority of respondents (97%) had previously received prescriptions for methadone, and thus the data reflects the experience and understanding of experienced methadone users. Notably, 66% of pre leaflet respondents realised methadone alone would not overcome their dependence, and only about 10% expected the treatment to be without difficulty.

The questionnaire results showed that the clients' knowledge of methadone was better than might have been anticipated, thus reducing the potential educational value of the leaflet to this group. One important benefit to the clients was the fact that many of them learned of the advantage of the drug being able to stabilise the habit and also that it was long-acting.

Overall, the PIL devised for this study was acceptable for those it targeted. However, insufficient information was provided on methadone's side effects, the concomitant use of alcohol, the need for careful oral hygiene, and the arrangements necessary for overseas travel. Future editions could be improved by the inclusion of a section on the possible physical effects of taking methadone such as weight gain, excessive sweating and suppression of cough reflex. Finally, it might be useful to include a paragraph on "Helping your pharmacist to help you". Such a booklet would be useful to pharmacists, drug workers and prescribers.

REFERENCES

1. Maddock DH. *Drug Abuse – A guide for pharmacists*. London: The Pharmaceutical Press; 1987.
2. Royal Pharmaceutical Society of Great Britain. Policy Statement: Pharmaceutical services for drug misusers. *The Pharmaceutical Journal* 1991; 247: 223.
3. Phillips GT, Gossop M, Bradley B. The influence of psychological factors on the opiate withdrawal syndrome. *British Journal of Psychiatry* 1986; 149: 235-238.
4. Green L, Gossop M. Effects of information on the opiate withdrawal syndrome. *British Journal of Addiction* 1988; 83: 305-309.
5. Goldsmith DS, Hunt DE, Lipton DS, Strug DL. Methadone Folklore: Beliefs about side effects and their impact on treatment. *Human Organisation* 1984; 43: 330-340.
6. Hermann F, Herxheimer A, Lionel NDW. Package inserts for prescribed medicines: What minimum information do patients need? *British Medical Journal* 1978; 2: 1132-5.
7. Owens DJ, Rees T, Parry-Langdon N. "All those in favour": Computerised Trade Union Membership. Lists as Sampling Frames for Postal Surveys. *Sociological Review* 1993; 41: 141-152.
8. Blum K. Methadone and other maintenance drugs; Side effects observed in patients during chronic methadone maintenance treatment. In: *Handbook of Abusable Drugs*. New York: Gardner Press; 1984, p108.
9. Gossop M, Eiser JR, Ward E. The addicts' perception of their own drug taking: implications for the treatment of drug dependence. *Addictive Behaviors* 1982; 7: 189-194.
10. Stastny D, Potter M. Alcohol abuse by patients undergoing methadone treatment programmes. *British Journal of Addiction* 1991; 86: 307-310.

CHAPTER ELEVEN

PROVIDING DRUG INJECTORS WITH EASIER ACCESS TO STERILE INJECTING EQUIPMENT

A description of a pharmacy based scheme

Neil McKeganey and Marina Barnard

INTRODUCTION

In an attempt at limiting the spread of HIV infection among injecting drug users, a range of mechanisms were initiated in the UK with the aim of providing easier access to sterile injecting equipment. Despite a good deal of controversy[1,2] public health policy makers have adopted a pragmatic approach to the problem of drug addiction arguing that abstinence, although a laudable goal, is not always possible or even desired by drug injectors.[3] In response to this, it has been widely accepted that those individuals who are unwilling or unable to stop injecting should at least be provided with means of obtaining sterile injecting equipment. These means range from the Government sponsored needle exchange schemes and the relaxation of constraints upon pharmacists selling injecting equipment, to the provision of injecting equipment by general practitioners, and the use of outreach workers to provide injecting equipment to drug injectors not in contact with treatment agencies.

Although the official needle exchange schemes have been extensively researched by Stimson and his colleagues[4,5] and others[6,7] there is only limited information on the operation of other mechanisms used to provide injecting equipment to injecting drug users. This is regrettable since building up a detailed picture of each of the various different mechanisms for providing sterile injecting equipment might better enable the tailoring of individual schemes to the needs of drug injectors and service providers in a local area.[8] Such information is of as much value to services designed specifically for the provision and exchange of needles and syringes (e.g. needle exchanges) as it is to pharmacists or detached workers who take on the work of providing injecting equipment.

In this chapter we describe the operation of one scheme for providing injecting equipment, namely a retail pharmacy operating within an area of Glasgow where drug injecting is widespread. Before looking in detail at the operation of the pharmacy it will be helpful to briefly provide some background information on drug injecting in Glasgow, on the wider study from which the data presented here are drawn, and the methods of collecting data on the work of the pharmacy.

BACKGROUND INFORMATION

Glasgow has a population of approximately 950,000 of whom 5000 were estimated to be injecting drug users in 1984.[9] More recently, Frischer *et al.*[10] have estimated that there may now be as many as 9424 injectors resident within the city. Despite recent research which has identified high levels of needle and syringe sharing amongst drug injectors in the city,[11,12] HIV infection remains relatively low. Glasgow is one of the cities participating in the WHO initiated cross-national study of drug injectors and HIV infection; analysis of the first year of data collection has identified an HIV prevalence figure of 1.4% for locally resident injectors.[13]

In the early 1980s Glasgow, along with many other British cities,[4] seems to have undergone a local epidemic of heroin use, much of which was concentrated in the poorest parts of the city. The pharmacy described in this paper is situated in one of those areas. Some idea of the extent of drug injecting in this area can be gained from the fact that over the last 3 years the pharmacist has been regularly selling between 3000-4000 sets of needles and syringes per month.

In 1981 this area was designated by the local authority as an "area for priority treatment" because of its markedly poor social and physical condition. In the 1981 census, unemployment among 16-24 year-olds was over 50%. Low income and unemployment are characteristic of many of the households. Numbers of single parents and large households are higher than average for the region, and 93% of households are without a car. In essence it is an area of multiple social deprivation.

From 1988 to 1991 a detailed sociological study of the area concentrating on drug injectors HIV-related risk behaviour was carried out. Methodologically this study has involved a combination of direct observation of drug injectors on the streets and in informal gatherings and semi-structured interviews carried out in a wide range of treatment settings. We have previously reported on such topics as the nature, extent and social meaning of needle and syringe sharing,[11,14] the nature and extent of the overlap between injecting drug users and female and male prostitution,[15,16] drug injectors experiences of HIV[14] and the knowledge and attitudes of young people living in an area where drug injecting is widespread.[17] Data for this chapter in particular was gained through a combination of direct observational work within the pharmacy over a 6-month period along with semi-structured interviews with staff and a sample of 102 clients purchasing injecting equipment. We have already reported data gained from these client interviews[11].

In the next section we will look at various aspects of the pharmacy's operation.

THE PHARMACY SCHEME

Location

The pharmacy is located on the main shopping street running through the housing scheme and is open 6 days a week from 9.00 am to 6.00 pm. The area immediately adjacent to the pharmacy is a well known meeting point for drug injectors. One of the benefits of being in such close proximity to the local drug culture is the accessibility of the pharmacy to local drug injectors. The pharmacy exists very much on the territory of the local people. At a simple level this means that the drug injectors do not have to travel very far to purchase their injecting equipment. Whilst this might seem a rather insignificant point, in fact many of the drug injectors we interviewed, and indeed, many local people in general were very territorial and were often reluctant to travel to other parts of the city. In addition, local drug injectors would make reference to rivalries with young people in neighbouring areas which could influence their preparedness to travel to other parts of the city:

> "I would not go down to the needle exchange because I'm too well known in X area and there'd be trouble."

Similar views were expressed by attenders at the nearby needle exchange in explaining their equivalent reluctance to attend the pharmacy. Proximity to the local drug using cultures then, both afforded access to some individuals and limited access to others.

It would be incorrect to suppose that there were no other costs associated with the location of the pharmacy. The pharmacy staff, for example, were local to the area and many of the drug injectors were familiar to them, some indeed, had grown up alongside their own children. Staff working in a setting that was regularly attended by large numbers of injecting drug users could not easily ignore the reality of widespread drug use. This would, on occasion, provoke a good deal of anxiety as to the possible future for their own adolescent sons and daughters.

Shona, one of the assistants, looked out of the window watching her sons walking up the main street "I don't like it, them just stoatin' (walking) about aimlessly". She then expounded "It's no' as if they don't know people that do it (take drugs), they grew up wi' them, they were at school wi' the ones that are doin' it, so it's no' as if they're strangers".

The Sale of Injecting Equipment

Providing drug injectors with the means to inject safely, and thereby reduce their risks of becoming HIV positive, was the *raison d'etre* behind the pharmacist's decision to begin selling sterile injecting equipment. To have denied drug injectors access to sterile equipment would, the pharmacist felt, have been to deny one of the central needs of many of the young people living in the area.

The policy of charging a small sum for injecting equipment (39p) arose first and foremost from the fact that the pharmacy is a retail environment. However, the policy of charging was felt to be important in other less tangible respects. According to the pharmacist this policy provided staff with a greater degree of control over drug injectors than would have been the case had staff been operating a free service. It enabled them to curb the disruptive behaviour that occasionally surfaced. In addition, the pharmacist also reported that as a result of charging he was able to provide a range of items such as sterile dressing and non-prescription medication for the treatment of injection site abscesses free of charge to drug injectors. There were many occasions during our observational work within the pharmacy when these items were provided in this way.

A minority of individuals interviewed within the pharmacy did comment unfavourably on the fact of having to pay for their injecting equipment:

"Both he and Mick complained about the cost of needles from the chemist saying that it was a 'real rip off'".

This view may have been based in part on reports in the local press to the effect that the issue of free distribution was being discussed by local service providers. However, the majority of individuals interviewed within the pharmacy regarded the sale of injecting equipment as par for the course. Indeed, few begrudged having to purchase their injecting equipment as they could remember a time when regular access to sterile needles and syringes was extremely difficult. Many spoke of previously having stolen injecting equipment from hospitals. The following comment is perhaps illustrative of a past lack of availability of clean needles and syringes:

"In the old days you had to pay half a Tem (Temgesic) for a hit, a set of works was like a bit of gold, you guarded them well".

Nevertheless, it must be recognized that even a minimum charge might act as a disincentive to some individuals regularly purchasing sterile injecting equipment. The scope for this is clearly apparent in the field note extract below which describes one individual's attempts to generate enough money to pay for her drug use.

> "As I came back into the chemist Maddie called me over asking me if I'd give her 30p. I said I only had 3p (true enough). She said she'd take it anyway. She was standing with a boy, both trying to tap people for money. Maddie said "I just need another £2.50 and that'll be me, one Tem (Temgesic), that's all". She'd been trying to raise the money since 1.00 pm. Her mother had given her £1.00 and she'd not been able to add to it since. While talking she suddenly saw a woman she knew and left saying "I'm gonnae tap Mrs A for 20p, see you after"".

It is relatively easy to see how this situation might result in the shared use of someone else's equipment in preference to begging the additional money for a sterile needle and syringe.

The Return of Non-Sterile Injecting Equipment

In most of the discussions surrounding the issue of providing sterile injecting equipment, concern has been expressed over the dangers associated with increases in the number of discarded needles and syringes. It is largely for this reason that emphasis has been placed (within the Government sponsored schemes) on the exchange of used injecting equipment for sterile needles and syringes.

At the time of this research within the pharmacy, there was no mechanism for the exchange of injecting equipment. The pharmacist felt that it would be potentially dangerous for his staff to receive possibly infected equipment within an often highly crowded retail environment. Similarly, he was also concerned as to the risks of having a disposable sharps container in a situation where young children were also present. The pharmacist's concern may not be unusual in this respect since a report on community pharmacists showed that most were unwilling to have sharps containers on the premises for the disposal of used injecting equipment.[18] As an alternative, needle clippers and small, rigid plastic containers for the safe disposal of used needles and syringes (Glenrothes Telescopes) were provided free of charge to those individuals purchasing injecting equipment. The possible dangers of accepting the return of drug injecting equipment were made clear during the time that one of us worked in the nearby needle exchange:

> "I asked him if he had any needles to return. He nodded and I got the box for him. As I held it out, he rather carelessly flung them into it. One of the needles missed and very nearly stuck into my thumb. I was quite disconcerted by this".

Such dangers existed within a setting specifically designed for the exchange of injecting equipment. Within the context of an often crowded retail pharmacy, the potential for such dangers might be even greater.

Counselling and Referral

There were occasions within the pharmacy when the pharmacist was able to provide advice, counselling and referral to those drug injectors in need.

> "Jai came into the pharmacy with a girl whose hand was swollen up. They asked if the pharmacist could help them, he took her to one side of the shop and cleaned and dressed the wound for her as well as advising her to see her GP with it".

However, since there was no part of the shop designated as a treatment area, advice had to be provided alongside the other work of the pharmacy, where time, and the demands of other customers, allowed. Additionally it would have been very difficult for the pharmacist to have initiated discussions in relation to sexual risk-taking. Indeed, even if a treatment area had been available it might still have been very difficult for the pharmacist to have raised such a topic with individuals who were primarily visiting the shop in order to purchase injecting equipment. This problem has been noted elsewhere in settings which do not have issues of sex and sexuality specifically on the agenda.[17]

Similarly, although on occasion the pharmacist would quite literally take a drug injector requiring treatment to the hospital, this would involve a major disruption to the work of the pharmacy and could, therefore, only happen in exceptional circumstances.

> This afternoon when I went into the shop the pharmacist told me that Mike (drug injector) had been in asking if the pharmacist could arrange for him to see a drug counsellor. The pharmacist said that he had been telephoning around agencies that afternoon. He added that on a previous occasion Mike had come into the shop with the worst leg abscesses he had ever seen and that he had taken him up to the hospital casualty to have them seen to.

Style of Working: The Use and Abuse of a Personal Relationship.

Although the restrictions on pharmacists selling needle and syringes have been relaxed since 1986[19] the decision as to whether or not to sell injecting equipment has been left largely to the discretion of individual pharmacists. There are relatively few guidelines as to how the sale of injecting equipment to injecting drug users should proceed. Individual pharmacist's have had to devise their own style of working and determine individual policies on such items as the numbers of needles and syringes they are prepared to provide to each individual and the minimum age at which they are prepared to provide equipment. Determining these policies in relation to the provision of injecting equipment can be a source of some considerable anxiety for pharmacy staff. The pharmacist we observed, for example, described the process of selling injecting equipment as akin to "walking a tightrope". Part of this feeling was rooted in the need to balance the objectives of being sufficiently friendly and open with the many drug injectors visiting the shop, whilst at the same time being sufficiently firm to curb the more socially disruptive aspects of their behaviour. Equally there was the need to balance the pharmacist's individual belief in the importance of providing injecting equipment with the sometimes critical views expressed on occasion by pharmacy colleagues and customers.

The range of difficult behaviours that staff had to contend with were fairly broad. Some drug injectors would shoplift items from within the pharmacy, others would demand immediate service from the pharmacist. Some would request injecting equipment with the promise of future payment and others would ask for the loan of small amounts of money. Events of this type undoubtedly increased the pressure on all the staff within the pharmacy. Of greater concern than all of these however, were those occasions when drug injectors would seek to persuade the pharmacist to sell or otherwise provide them with prescription only drugs. Such requests were seen by the pharmacist as an unwelcome attempt at compromising the personal relationship he had established with the individual drug injector and his own professional standards:

> The pharmacist related how a drug injector regular to the shop had asked him if he could help him out. He said that he would be getting a prescription for Temazepam later on and would the pharmacist give him some now to tide him over? The pharmacist had refused. "I told him firmly. He's got to know that I can't just give him tablets. You want to help but not in that way, that's absolutely out of the question."

Given the preponderance of drugs within the pharmacy it is probably inevitable that individual drug injectors would make such requests at some point. As a result, however, the pharmacist was constantly having to restate the standards of acceptable behaviour within the pharmacy in order to guard against the possibility of being manipulated by certain individual drug injectors:

> During the afternoon the pharmacist gave eight sets of injecting equipment out to people on promise of future payment. He said he felt like he was becoming the needle exchange. The shop assistant commented adversely on it saying she felt they were getting really cheeky. The pharmacist replied "I've been too lenient, now I'll have to screw the nut and get things back in order again".

DISCUSSION

Within the context of an agreed policy as to the importance of providing drug injectors with easier access to sterile injecting equipment, community pharmacies clearly represent one possible distribution point. However, the mechanics of distributing sterile injecting equipment through pharmacies have yet to be clearly outlined.

In this chapter we have described one such scheme. In terms of the numbers of needles and syringes regularly provided over the last 2 years, this scheme has been very successful. Part of that success has to do with the location of the pharmacy within an area where drug injecting is widespread, along with the pharmacist and the staff's capacity to develop a user-friendly style of working. Nevertheless, the contact with large numbers of injecting drug users established as a result of the policy of selling injecting equipment also involved certain costs. Staff have had to cope with a range of behaviours which whilst not unique to injecting drug users have certainly increased as a result of the numbers of drug injectors now visiting the shop.

In certain respects drug injectors are no different from any of the other customers a pharmacist and his or her staff have to deal with. However, in certain other respects drug injectors can be very different; they can attend the shop whilst experiencing the effects of drug withdrawal and be irritable and impatient as a result; they can present in a confused and uncoordinated manner whilst experiencing the effects of recent drug use; they can request treatment for abscesses, or present with a range of infections including HIV and hepatitis. In addition they can attempt to steal items or try to persuade the pharmacist to sell them drugs.

Encouraging the participation of pharmacists in needle and syringe provision to injecting drug users is clearly an important step in the wider policy of reducing needle and syringe sharing and HIV spread. It cannot be assumed, however, that pharmacy staff already possess the requisite skills for coping with this population. It is very important that those schemes that are set up remain stable and operational. Perhaps the worst arrangement of all is one where pharmacists opt in and out of providing injecting equipment depending on the shifting nature of their individual experiences. However, this is very likely to occur in a situation where individual pharmacists are left on their own to resolve the mechanics of needle and syringe provision. Adequate account needs to be taken of the complex operational and personal issues involved in work of this kind. A strong case can be made for ensuring that pharmacists and their staff are able to draw upon the experience of other pharmacists working in this area. In addition, there is a need to ensure that those pharmacists who have opted to participate in such schemes have adequate back-up and support from relevant agencies.

ACKNOWLEDGEMENT

The research on which this paper is based was funded by the Economic and Social Research Council as part of their AIDS programme. In addition we would like to acknowledge the support of Harry Watson in this study. The Centre for Drug Misuse Research is funded by the Chief Scientist Office of the Scottish Home and Health Department. The opinions expressed in this paper are not necessarily those of the Scottish Home and Health Department.

In order to maintain confidentiality we have altered individual's names and certain minor biographical details.

This is a modified version of an article that was first published in *The British Journal of Addiction* 1992; 87: 987-992.

REFERENCES

1. Farid B. AIDS and drug addiction needle exchange schemes: a step in the dark. *Journal of the Royal Society of Medicine* 1988; 81: 375-376.
2. Cook CCH. Syringe exchange (letter). *The Lancet* 1987; i: 920-921.
3. Strang J. Changing injecting practices: blunting the needle habit. *British Journal of Addiction* 1988; 83: 237-239.
4. Stimson GV. The war on heroin: British policy and the international trade in illicit drugs. In: Dorn N, South N. eds. *A land fit for heroin: Drug policies, Prevention, and Practice*. London: Macmillan; 1987.
5. Stimson GV. Syringe exchange programmes for injecting drug users. *AIDS* 1989; 3: 253-260.
6. Hart G, Carvell A, Woodward N, Johnson AM, Williams P, Parry JV. Evaluation of needle exchange in central London: behaviour change and anti-HIV status over one year. *AIDS* 1989; 3: 261-265.
7. Hartgers C, Buning EC, Van Santen GW, Verster AD, Coutinho RA. The impact of the needle and syringe exchange programme in Amsterdam on injecting risk behaviour. *AIDS* 1989; 3: 571-576.
8. Koli HS, Goldberg D. Intravenous drug misuse: has the pharmacist a role? *AIDS News Supplement Weekly Report* 1987; CDS 87/42, No. A29.
9. Haw S. *Drug Problems in Greater Glasgow: Report of the SCODA Fieldwork Survey in Greater Glasgow Health Board*. Glasgow: SCODA; 1985.
10. Frischer M, Bloor M, Finlay A, Goldberg D, Green S, Haw S, McKeganey N, Platt S. A new method of estimating the prevalence of injecting drug use in an urban population: results from a Scottish city. *International Journal of Epidemiology* 1992; 20: 997-1000.
11. McKeganey N, Barnard M, Watson H. HIV-related risk behaviour among a non-clinic sample of injecting drug users. *The British Journal of Addiction* 1989; 84: 1481-1490.
12. McKeganey N. Drug abuse in the community: needle sharing and the risks of HIV infection. In: Cunningham-Burley S, McKeganey N. eds. *Readings in Medical Sociology*. London: Routledge; 1989.

13. Haw S, Frischer M, Covell R *et al.* HIV infection and risk behaviour among injecting drug users in Glasgow. *AIDS News Supplement Weekly Report 91/320 A210.* Scotland; 1991.

14. McKeganey N. Being positive: drug injectors' experiences of HIV infection. *The British Journal of Addiction* 1990; 85: 1113-1124.

15. McKeganey N, Barnard M, Bloor M. A comparison of HIV related risk behaviour and risk reduction between female street working prostitutes and male rent boys in Glasgow. *Sociology of Health and Illness* 1990; 12: 274-292.

16. McKeganey N, Barnard M, Bloor M, Leyland A. Injecting drug use and female street working prostitution in Glasgow. *AIDS* 1990; 4:1153-1155.

17. Barnard M, McKeganey N. Adolescents, sex and injecting drug use: risks for HIV infection. *AIDS Care* 1990; 2: 103-116.

18. Glanz A, Byrne C, Jackson P. Role of community pharmacies in prevention of AIDS among injecting drug misusers: findings of a survey in England and Wales. *British Medical Journal* 1989; 299: 1076-1079.

19. Council of the Pharmaceutical Society of Great Britain. Sale of hypodermic syringes and needles. *The Pharmaceutical Journal* 1986; 236: 205.

CHAPTER TWELVE

ACCOUNTING FOR VARIATION IN DRUG THERAPY

Clinical uncertainty, professional autonomy and the issue of rational prescribing

Peter Davis

INTRODUCTION

This chapter addresses the question of variation in medical practice. It does so with particular reference to drug utilisation and to patterns of prescribing. Clinical uncertainty and professional autonomy are identified as the two key factors contributing to variation in medical practice and, by extension, to variability in prescribing behaviour. After a preliminary review of the broader field, the chapter presents a case study of prescribing variation in a sample of New Zealand general practitioners. The overall pattern of prescribing is similar to that reported in comparable studies of general practice in the United Kingdom and ambulatory care in the United States. The variations between practitioners are marked and are only in part explained by differences in morbidity, attesting to the existence of distinct practitioner styles or prescribing "signatures". There remains an important role for pharmacists in encouraging rational patterns of drug therapy.

IS MEDICINE INTERNATIONAL?

In her book "Medicine and Culture", the journalist Lynn Payer asks the question in the title of her opening chapter, "Is Medicine International?", and then goes on to give the reader sufficient detail on the variation in the medical cultures of France, Germany, England and the United States to suggest that, at the very least, we cannot easily dismiss the notion that there exist quite distinct national styles of medical practice.[1]

The Germans, for example, dose themselves liberally with drugs for heart disease and show great concern about low blood pressure, a diagnosis that is scarcely recognised in Anglo-American medicine. They have a vast number of drugs on the market, many drugs are in combination form, they go to the doctor frequently (on average about once a month), and they receive more prescription items than most. While some preparations are used very freely – like digitalis – others such as antibiotics are used much more sparingly.

For the French, by contrast, the liver is the all-important organ. Many conditions are attributed to it, from the liver "crisis" – generally a severe migraine – through headaches and gastrointestinal upsets to painful menstruation and general fatigue. There are many different medications for the liver on the French market, and the consumption of drugs for the treatment of the digestive system is high. Tonics are widely used, there is a greater reliance on homeopathic and other "gentle medicines", and suppositories are more frequently used for medication. There is also a much higher use of peripheral vasodilators, drugs greatly restricted in use elsewhere.

The difference between the British and American traditions of medical practice, as Payer sees it, is in the parsimony, economy and conservative attitude to treatment of the one and the highly-interventionist, even aggressive, disposition that characterises the American approach to therapy from birth through to death. This is reflected in a high use of screening and diagnostic tests, a preference for surgery over drugs, and, when drugs are used, higher doses of generally more potent preparations.

These vignettes are impressionistic, but nevertheless they are based on documented evidence and they provide great insight into different national styles of medical practice. The notion that there might be distinct medical "cultures" is supported by the evidence on variations between European countries in rates of medical contact and patterns of prescribing. From this data there appear to be two broad medical "cultures" in Western Europe. Germany aside, in Northwestern Europe and the English-speaking world people generally attend the doctor less frequently and receive fewer prescription items. In the Mediterranean countries, and Belgium, the opposite is true.[2]

EXPLAINING VARIABILITY

There is evidence, therefore, that there are systematic differences between countries in styles of medical practice, including the level and pattern of drug usage. These can be plausibly related to aspects of culture and to the organisation and funding of health care. The question then still remains – if modern medicine is based on much the same scientific premises about the body and its functioning, how can such striking differences in treatment patterns result? To say that culture and the delivery system are influential, is merely to push the question back one step further – why is the practice of modern medicine susceptible to the influence of such factors, given its firm grounding in the biomedical sciences?

The answer to this question is twofold. Firstly, while biomedicine is indeed at the cutting edge of modern laboratory science, with a powerfully predictive and conceptually sophisticated body of knowledge, its actual application in the treatment of patients is strongly influenced by elements of human judgement and contingency. Although some advances have been made in applying the epidemiological and social sciences to evaluating the application of different treatments in the clinical setting - for example, by using Randomised Controlled Trials (RCTs)[3] – there still remains considerable uncertainty, and thus room for discretionary judgement, in medical practice.[4]

What this "uncertainty" hypothesis does not explain is why, for those treatments about which there is virtual unanimity, considerable variation remains, and why, for those treatments that have long been established as either ineffective, unnecessarily costly, or even harmful, practitioners often fail to respond to the evidence. The answer seems to lie in the doctrine of clinical freedom – the right to make an independent professional judgement – which, while it maximises the opportunities for a flexible and appropriate response to the special and unique characteristics of each patient, serves also to protect patterns of practice that may be outmoded and that may have no justification other than tradition or personal preference to commend them.[5]

Why Investigate Variability?

Clinical uncertainty and professional autonomy, therefore, when combined with cultural and organisational factors, provide the most potent explanation for variability in medical practice. But it might well be asked, why investigate such variations? Certainly, such data challenges the received view of medicine as a homogeneous and scientifically based activity, but what else does it achieve?

There are three reasons. First, the range of variability may include patterns of practice that are actually harmful. These are not generally or routinely acted upon in the course of the profession's own systems of internal review unless a practitioner is impaired in some way, say, by drugs, alcohol, or a psychiatric problem.[6] Secondly, governments have become much more concerned about the costs of health care and the effective allocation of resources, and are increasingly moving to impose various controls and encourage the evaluation of medical intervention.[7]

Finally, there is the question of fairness. One of the reasons that governments are involved in the funding and provision of health care is to ensure that such resources are available on the basis of need rather than ability to pay. If practitioners are allocating resources in ways that fail to accord with accepted requirements of need, then a fundamental goal of public policy is not being fulfilled.[8]

While the goals of public policy provide the crucial motivation for research into variability, it is the findings of such research that generate the insights into potential areas of intervention. Hence, depending on whether cultural, organisational, informational or professional factors are shown to be important, so a range of possible approaches open up – education, regulation, economic instruments, administrative review, self-regulation, and so on.[9]

METHODS

Sources of Variation

An initial hypothesis in considering variations in medical practice is that such variability reflects actual differences in the *need* for treatment. In most cases such an explanation is rarely a sufficient one, but failure to take morbidity into account – either directly, if the data is available, or with sociodemographic and epidemiological indicators – can produce seriously misleading interpretations. One practical consequence of this is the importance placed on standardising comparisons by age and gender.[10]

A further hypothesis that has already been extensively canvassed is that of *cultural* difference. At the international level, for example, once age structure has been taken into account, differences in medical culture would appear to be the most plausible explanation for variation, along with health system factors and resource availability. The concept of medical culture as used here refers to differences in the way in which people respond to symptoms, make sense of them, and seek to act upon them. Although more usually considered in the context of lay responses, this notion is also helpful in thinking about the pattern of professional responses.[11]

The explanation that has most readily come to hand is one that has been couched in terms of *health system* factors, such as the availability of resources and the way doctors are paid. Within a country there is likely to be much more variation in the distribution of resources than in patterns of reimbursement. There will also be other specifically organisational factors, such as the way medical practice is organised, the training and specialty of doctors, and the distribution of other health personnel.[12]

The remaining two broad categories of substantive explanation that have been discussed relate to information and to clinical autonomy. In a sense clinical autonomy is invariate; it is the condition of medical practice. While there may be other factors of a professional character – such as continuing medical education, the potential for peer review in the group practice setting – the key issue seems to be an informational one; that is, the level of uncertainty associated with the particular intervention, the information that is available to practitioners, and the way in which it might influence *clinical* decisions[13].

The final source of variation is not substantively important, but nevertheless is a vital consideration in research in this area. In interpreting differences in rates of intervention it is always possible that the observed variation is either wholly or in part a function of *error*. Much statistical acumen is devoted to modelling the effects of random errors and seeking to account for their significance in explaining variability. Great effort is also expended in trying to ensure that data sources are complete and accurate.[10]

Levels of Aggregation

Typically, studies in this field are carried out at either the level of cross-national comparison, regional or "small area" statistics[14], or practitioner differences. If we take both the level at which the data is aggregated, and the different sources of variation, it is possible to compile a reasonably comprehensive check list of the kinds of explanation and the significance of the evidence derived from studies in different research settings (see Table 1).

At the level of *cross-national* comparison, research is less subject to random errors, but there are problems in gaining exactly comparable data sets and definitions. The types of factors that are most clearly involved in explaining variation in these comparisons are cultural and organisational.

Research *within* countries carried out at the level of key administrative areas is more subject to random error, but overcoming problems of accuracy and completeness in the data are more feasible. There are likely to be large differences between such areas in sociodemographic composition and in the availability and configuration of resources.

TABLE 1: Hypothesised impact of variation by level of aggregation
(after reference 10)

Sources of Variation	Levels of Aggregation		
	COUNTRIES	REGIONS	PRACTITIONERS
NEED	Small	Medium	Medium
CULTURAL	Large	Small	Small
HEALTH SYSTEM	Large	Medium	Small
CLINICAL	Small	Medium	Large
ERROR	Systematic	Random	Random

Comparisons *between* practitioners, by contrast, while particularly subject to random error because of the smaller numbers involved, are likely to maximise the influence of informational and organisational factors related to clinical work. After the influence of sociodemographic differences have been controlled, one might expect attributes of the practice setting and of the practitioner to have the most salient impact on the pattern of variation. It is with this level of practitioner variation that the illustrative case study is concerned[15].

THE NEW ZEALAND STUDY

The data are drawn from the Community Medical Care Survey (CoMedCa), a 1% sample of all weekday general practice office encounters in the Hamilton health district recorded over a twelve month period from February 1979. Ninety per cent of 128 doctors active in general practice in the area at the time co-operated, with a further loss of less than 8% of data collection weeks due to illness or other absence from practice. The study produced nearly 9,500 completed patient encounter records.

Each patient encounter record was filled out by the general practitioner at the time of contact and included age, gender, occupation, ethnic group, diagnosis, severity of condition and a full log of diagnostic, therapeutic and disposition activities.

Social class was coded from the occupational information and collapsed into manual and non-manual groupings. Ethnic affiliations were combined into two groups, Maori – the indigenous Polynesian people of New Zealand – and non-Maori. Diagnoses were grouped approximately according to chapter headings of the *International Classification of Diseases* (9th revision). For symptomatic conditions, severity was judged by the general practitioner as high, medium or low.

Information was collected on key practice and practitioner characteristics. Practitioner attributes that could be determined from available sources were age, country of qualification, and level of qualification, but not gender. Practice variables used were size, number of patients seen per day, area, and standard fee. A variable was also created for practitioner identity.

Data on four service activities was available: laboratory test orders, prescriptions, referrals, and request for follow up. Detailed analysis was carried out on prescribing activity, for which seven binary measures were constructed addressing volume (number of items prescribed, length of supply), prescription detail (generic specification, combination preparation), and therapeutic choice (three indicator drug categories). Where a drug was prescribed for one, two or three months, this was classified as "extended supply". A generic specification was defined as a non-proprietary description of a preparation, and combination drugs as preparations containing more than one active ingredient, each having a different therapeutic property. For the selected drugs three classes with a wide range of indications and/or disputable applications were identified; these were systemic antibiotics, analgesics, and psychotropics. In the case of multiple drug prescriptions scripts were classified into as many prescribing activity categories as required.

In order to assess the relative effects of different potential explanatory factors in the model, a multivariate analysis was required. Since the prescribing activity measures were not continuous in form, they were rendered as binary variables for the purposes of the analysis. The analysis was carried out using the GLM procedure within SAS. This procedure has the capacity to handle qualitative (classificatory) variables as predictors. It is also able to accommodate a variable with multiple classes or categories; in the case of "practitioner identity" each class represented a different doctor. Measures of association and estimates of effect are calculated from the component sums of squares. The unique contribution of a variable is given by the decrease in predictive power that occurs when that variable is removed from the analysis.

RESULTS

The focus of this study is variation in medical practice, and Table 2 addresses the distribution of four service activities among practitioners. For each service, practitioners were ranked according to their activity level and grouped into thirds (terciles). The difference in rates of service activity between upper and lower terciles is marked, generally lying approximately one standard deviation either side of the overall mean. In most cases this reflects practically a twofold

TABLE 2: Distribution of service activity levels: mean percentage of patients receiving service by practitioner tercile
(reproduced with permission from reference 15).

Doctor Tercile	Percentage of Patients Receiving Service			
	LAB. TEST	SCRIPT	REFERRAL	FOLLOW UP
UPPER	26.0	72.4	12.2	56.5
MIDDLE	14.7	63.4	7.2	42.2
LOWER	6.9	49.7	3.8	30.4
MEAN	15.9	61.8	7.7	43.0
(RANGE)	(1.1–48.8)	(30.6–82.4)	(0–20.1)	(15.1–78.3)

variation. The extreme ends of the range are strikingly discrepant. For example, practitioner orders for tests vary between 1% and nearly half of all patients seen. The upper limit for prescribing and follow up is about 80%.

Table 3 extends this analysis to the full range of prescribing activity measures, but only for that proportion of the sample – roughly 40% of encounters – for which a script has been written and for which there is a single diagnosis. This is in order to permit as close an alignment as possible between diagnosis and therapeutic choice. There is much the same shape to the distributions. Variation among individual practitioners is also marked, ranging from zero to 100% for two measures. Only for analgesics and psychotropics is the upper end of the range less than 50%, and this is largely because of the lower overall mean level of activity for these therapeutic classes.

TABLE 3: Distribution of prescribing activity: mean percentageof patients receiving service by practitioner tercile (single-diagnosis consultations only).

Practitioner Tercile	>1 Drug	Ext. Supply	Generic	Combination Drug	Antibiotic	Analgesic	Psychotropic
UPPER	56.6	71.8	35.8	58.3	52.6	20.7	12.3
MIDDLE	40.1	45.3	21.1	40.9	37.4	11.0	4.7
LOWER	23.8	27.2	9.1	26.2	22.8	3.8	0.5
OVERALL MEAN	40.2	48.1	22.0	41.8	37.6	11.8	5.8
(RANGE)	(0–77)	(0–100)	(0–52)	(0–100)	(0–72)	(0–35)	(0–20)

The particular interest of the current study is in the impact of various potential sources of variation on the pattern of prescribing. According to the model discussed in Table 1, in the analysis of practitioner variation, sociodemographic and epidemiological differences should be significant, but once these factors have been held constant, practice organisation and practitioner attributes could be expected to exert a significant effect.

An adequate assessment of this model can only be derived using multivariate techniques. This is addressed in Table 4 where classes of like attributes have been grouped and their effects pooled, with the percentage of variation explained expressed as a cumulative total for each grouping. This figure summarises the collective impact of a group of attributes on a given measure of prescribing activity. To take the last column for example: diagnosis accounts for 34.8% of the variation in the use of psychotropics, patient characteristics for less than 1%, and practitioner identity for 3.6%. For statistical reasons both practitioner identity and practitioner and practice attributes cannot be represented in the same table. For illustrative purposes, and for reasons of substantive interest, only the analysis involving practitioner identity is shown here.

TABLE 4: Determinants of prescribing activity: percentage of variation explained by practitioner identity, patient and diagnostic characteristics
(single-diagnosis consultations – only)

	>1 Drug	Ext. Supply	Generic	Combination Drug	Antibiotic	Analgesic	Psychotropic
DIAGNOSIS							
% VAR EXPL	6.7%	10.6%	1.6%	5.1%	22.4%	4.4%	34.8%
PATIENT CHARACTERISTICS							
% VAR EXPL	0.4%	1.3%	0.5%	0.7%	2.0%	0.7%	0.4%
PRACTITIONER IDENTITY							
% VAR EXPL	7.5%	13.7%	9.3%	6.8%	4.3%	5.9%	3.6%
FULL MODEL*							
% VAR EXPL	16.4%	35.8%	12.0%	14.1%	42.0%	11.7%	43.9%
(CORRELATION)	(0.41)	(0.60)	(0.35)	(0.38)	(0.65)	(0.34)	(0.66)

*The individual items of variation explained do not normally add up to the total explained by the model because of interaction effects.

Looking first at the total predictive power of the model – percentage of variance explained in the bottom row – only three measures show any substantial level of explanatory power – that is, Extended Supply (35.8%), Antibiotics (42.0%) and Psychotropics (43.9%) – and in these cases diagnosis and practitioner identity are the crucial factors, as they are throughout the table. In essence the identity of the practitioner is in aggregate as important a predictor as diagnosis, but it exerts a consistently weaker influence in the determination of therapeutic choice (the three indicator drugs).

In a result reported elsewhere, practitioner and practice attributes were substituted for practitioner identity in the analysis.[16] Again, diagnosis was important, but there were few instances where the cumulated effect of any non-diagnostic group of attributes amounted to more than 1%, except, again, for patient characteristics. To all intents and purposes the impact of organisational and professional factors on prescribing activity was negligible.

DISCUSSION

The current investigation confirms the existence of the marked variations reported elsewhere in service activity among general practitioners. Apart from laboratory tests, the overall rates of activity are quite comparable to levels recorded in a recent British study of urban general practice.[17] Particularly notable is the evidence of striking disparities in activity level between the upper and lower limits of the range.

This study has outlined prescribing patterns in a representative sample of general practice encounters using a range of measures of volume, script detail, and therapeutic choice. *Cross-national* differences in patterns of drug utilisation have been well documented for overall levels of consumption[18] and for specific categories such as antibiotics[19], antihypertensives[20,21], tranquillisers[22], and the treatment of diabetes[23,24] and cerebrovascular disease[25]. *Within* countries similar differences have been documented by population density[26], by region[27], by population age-sex structure[28], across hospitals[29] and other institutions[30], and across types of practice organisation and payment systems[31].

At first sight the results of the current study would seem to run counter to this literature on variation in drug utilisation and prescribing practice. Certainly the study confirms the existence of considerable variation among practitioners, but there seem to be few striking differences in patterns of practice when compared with results reported in comparable settings elsewhere for most of the seven measures of prescribing activity. Aside from the figures for antibiotics and compound preparations, which seem to be high, these results are broadly similar to the international benchmark data reported for the National Ambulatory Medical Care Survey in the United States.[32] Neither do these results seem too out of line with British figures.[16]

Nevertheless, this probably understates the total amount of variability because the denominator for the rates of drug utilisation in this study is the practice sample rather than the catchment population. This means that major potential sources of population variation have been omitted, such as social differences in the resort to medical care. In essence, therefore, this is a study of practice patterns – rather than population influences – and it appears that in aggregate these patterns are not unlike those reported for the United States and the United Kingdom.

What remains, however, is a much sharper picture of variation *within* a practice sample. While the cross-national differences in patterns of practice may be minor, there is marked within country variation in prescribing behaviour among practitioners. The prescribing variation recorded in this sample is on a par with the variability in the other measures of service activity. What accounts for this variation? The minimal impact of patient, practice, and practitioner attributes suggests that once the decision has been taken to write a prescription, the key clinical judgement is not influenced in a systematic way by such attributes. The prescribing decision seems to be a function of diagnosis, the clinical style of the practitioner, and a large, as yet unexplained, component of variation.

Only two of the indicator drugs and one measure of volume come anywhere close to a satisfactory level of prediction under the statistical model. Both diagnosis and practitioner identity account for significant levels of variation on practically every measure, with identity being more important for volume and script detail, and diagnosis for therapeutic choice.

Inconclusiveness on this score confirms the paucity of positive results in the literature. However, while identifiable practice and practitioner attributes do not seem to exert a significant systematic influence on prescribing patterns, there remains a strong indication in the present study that practitioners exhibit more or less distinct prescribing profiles or "signatures"[14] that invite further investigation.

IMPLICATIONS

The significance of prescribing variation is threefold. Firstly, doctors are essentially gatekeepers to treatment.[33] Secondly, their decisions commit anything up to 80% of all health care costs.[34] Thirdly, variability raises important questions about the quality and fairness of prescribing decisions.[35]

The prescribing decision is a complex one subject to a number of influences.[36] It is often made rapidly under conditions of clinical uncertainty in which key elements are the source of available information,[37,38] its acceptability[39] and its interpretation.[40]

A considerable amount of research has been carried out on interventions designed to change prescribing patterns.[41] It is evident that simple administrative remedies are, at best, a blunt instrument[42] and may frequently have harmful effects.[43] The most successful interventions are those that involve individualised instruction related to the clinical experience of the practitioner,[44] that take into account the attitudes and motivations of practitioners[45], and that are sustained over a period of time.[46] There are opportunities here for a fruitful and satisfying working relationship between doctors and pharmacists in enhancing rational patterns of prescribing.

ACKNOWLEDGEMENTS

This paper was written while I was on Sabbatical Leave from the University of Auckland and a Visiting Scholar at the Center for Health and Advanced Policy Studies, Boston University. I am grateful to both institutions for their support. Thanks for access to the consultation data are due to the CoMedCa team headed by Dr Ian Scott and funded by the Medical Research Council of New Zealand. My thanks also to Dr John Millar for assisting with the classification of the drugs and to Roy Lay Yee for the preparation of Tables 2,3 and 4.

REFERENCES

1. Payer L. *Medicine and Culture. Varieties of Treatment in the United States, England, West Germany, and France.* New York: Henry Holt and Company; 1988, pp157-192.
2. National Consumer Council. *Pharmaceuticals. A Consumer Prescription.* London: National Consumer Council; 1991, p24.
3. Cochrane AL. *Effectiveness and Efficiency: Random Reflections on Health Services.* London: Nuffield Hospital Provincial Trust; 1972.
4. Wennberg JE, Barnes BA, Zubkoff M. Professional uncertainty and the problem of supplier-induced demand. *Social Science and Medicine* 1982; 16: 811-824.
5. Evans RG. The dog in the night-time: Medical practice variations and health policy. In: Andersen TF and Mooney G eds. *The Challenge of Medical Practice Variations.* London: Macmillan; 1990, pp117-152.
6. Morrow C. The medicalization of professional self-governance: A sociological approach. In: Swazey J, Scher S eds. *Social Controls and the Medical Profession.* Boston MA: Eelgeschlager, Gunn and Hain; 1984, pp163-184.
7. Rutten FHR, Bonsel GJ. High cost technology in health care: a benefit or a burden? *Social Science and Medicine* 1992; 35: 567-577.
8. Bevan G. Equity and variability in modern health care. In: Andersen TF, Mooney G eds. *The Challenge of Medical Practice Variations.* London: Macmillan; 1990, pp76-94.
9. Davis P. Pharmaceuticals and public policy: Learning from the New Zealand experience. *Health Policy* 1993; 24: 259-272.
10. McPherson K. Why do variations occur? In: Andersen TF, Mooney G eds. *The Challenge of Medical Practice Variations* London: Macmillan; 1990, pp16-35.
11. Aaron HJ, Schwartz WB. *The Painful Prescription.* Washington DC: The Brookings Institute; 1984.
12. Wennberg JE, Fowler F. A test of consumer contribution to small area variations in health care delivery. *Journal of the Maine Medical Association* 1977; 68: 275-279.
13. Mulley AG. Medical decision making and practice variation. In: Andersen TF, Mooney G eds. *The Challenge of Medical Practice Variations.* London: Macmillan; 1990, pp59-75.
14. Wennberg JE, Gittelsohn A. Variations in medical care among small areas. *Scientific American* 1982; 246: 120-134.
15. Davis PB, Yee RL. Patterns of care and professional decision making in a New Zealand general practice sample. *New Zealand Medical Journal* 1990; 103: 309-312.
16. Davis PB, Yee RL, Millar J. Accounting for medical variation: The case of prescribing activity in a New Zealand general practice sample. *Social Science and Medicine* (in press).

17. Wilkin D, Hallam L, Leavey R, Metcalfe D. *Anatomy of Urban General Practice.* London: Tavistock; 1987.
18. Szuba TJ. International comparison of drug consumption: impact of prices. *Social Science and Medicine* 1986; 22: 1019-1026.
19. Harvey K. Antibiotic use in Australia. *Australian Prescriber* 1988; 11: 74-77.
20. Baksaas I. Patterns in drug utilization – national and international aspects: antihypertensive drugs. *Acta Medica Scandinavica* [Suppl] 1983; 683: 59-66.
21. Griffiths K, McDevitt DG, Andrew M, Baksaas I, Helgeland A, Jervell J, Lunde PK, Oyduin K, Agenas I, Bergmar W. Therapeutic traditions in Northern Ireland, Norway and Sweden: II Hypertension. *European Journal of Clinical Pharmacology* 1986; 30: 521-525.
22. Balter MB, Levine J, Manheimer DI. Cross-national study of the extent of anti-anxiety/sedative drug use. *New England Journal of Medicine* 1974; 290: 769-774.
23. Griffiths K, McDevitt DG, Andrew M, Baksaas I, Helgeland A, Jervell J, Lunde PK, Oyduin K, Agenas I, Bergmar W. Therapeutic traditions in Northern Ireland, Norway and Sweden: I Diabetes. *European Journal of Clinical Pharmacology* 1986; 30: 513-519.
24. Stika L. Patterns in drug utilization – national and international aspects: antidiabetic drugs. *Acta Medica Scandinavica* [Suppl] 1983; 683: 53-57.
25. Spagnoli A, Tognoni G, Darmansjah I, Laporte JR, Vrhovac B, Treacher DF, Warlow CP. A multinational comparison of drug treatment in patients with cerebrovascular disease. *European Neurology* 1985; 24: 4-12.
26. Gabe J, Williams P. Rural tranquillity? Urban-rural differences in tranquilliser prescribing. *Social Science and Medicine* 1986; 22: 1059-1066.
27. Christiansen T, Pedersen KM, Harvald B, Rasmussen K, Jorgensen J, Svarer C. An investigation of the effect of regional variation in the treatment of hypertension. *Social Science and Medicine* 1989; 28: 131-139.
28. Forster DP, Frost CE. Use of regression analysis to explain the variation in prescribing rates and costs between family practitioner committees. *British Journal of General Practice* 1991; 41: 67-71.
29. Hjort PF, Homen J, Waaler HT. Relation between drug utilization and morbidity patterns: antihypertensive drugs. *Acta Medica Scandinavica* [Suppl] 1984; 683: 89-93.
30. Nolan L, O'Malley K. The need for a more rational approach to drug prescribing for elderly people in nursing homes. *Age and Ageing* 1989; 18: 52-56.
31. Greenfield S, Nelson EC, Zubkoff M, Manning W, Rogers W, Kravitz RL, Keller A, Tarlov AR, Ware JE. Variations in resource utilization among medical specialties and systems of care. Results from the medical outcomes study. *Journal of the American Medical Association* 1992; 267: 1624-1630.
32. National Center for Health Statistics. *Highlights of drug utilization in office practice: National Ambulatory Medical Care Survey 1985.* Hyattsville MD: Public Health Service, USDHHS; 1987. (Advanced Data from Vital and Health Statistics, no. 134).
33. Christensen DB, Bush PJ. Drug prescribing: patterns, problems and proposals. *Social Science and Medicine* 1981; 15: 243-255.

34. Eisenberg JM, Williams SV. Cost containment and changing physicians' practice behavior. *Journal of the American Medical Association* 1981; 241: 2195-2201.
35. Carrin G. Drug prescribing: A discussion of its variability and (ir)rationality. *Health Policy* 1987; 7: 73-94.
36. Bradley CP. Decision making and prescribing patterns – a literature review. *Family Practice* 1991; 8: 276-287.
37. Avorn J, Chen M, Hartley R. Scientific vs. commercial sources of influence on physician prescribing behavior. *American Journal of Medicine* 1982; 73: 4-8.
38. Bower AD, Burkett GL. Family physicians and generic drugs: A study of recognition, information sources, prescribing attitudes, and practices. *Journal of Family Practice* 1987; 24: 612-616.
39. Christensen DB, Wertheimer AI. Sources of information and influence on new drug prescribing among physicians in an HMO. *Social Science and Medicine* 1979; 13: 313-322.
40. Soumerai SB, Avorn J. Principles of educational outreach ('academic detailing') to improve clinical decision making. *Journal of the American Medical Association* 1990; 263: 549-556.
41. Wyatt TD, Reilly PM, Morrow NC, Passmore CM. Short-lived effects of a formulary on anti-infective prescribing – the need for continuing peer review? *Family Practice* 1992; 9: 461-465.
42. Soumerai SB, Ross-Degnan D, Gortmaker S, Avorn J. Withdrawing payment for non-scientific drug therapy: intended and unexpected effects of a large scale natural experiment. *Journal of the American Medical Association* 1990; 263: 831-839.
43. Soumerai SB, Ross-Degnan D, Avorn J, McLaughlin TJ, Choodnovskiy I. Effects of Medicaid drug-payment limits on admission to hospitals and nursing homes. *New England Journal of Medicine* 1991; 325: 1072-1077.
44. Manning PR, Lee PV, Clintworth WA, et al. Changing prescribing practices through individual continuing education. *Journal of the American Medical Association* 1986; 256: 230-232.
45. Schwartz RK, Soumerai SB, Avorn J. Physician motivations for nonscientific drug prescribing. *Social Science and Medicine* 1989; 28: 577-582.
46. Feely J, Chan R, Cocoman L. Impact of a hospital formulary on prescribing habits and drug costs. *Irish Medical Journal* 1987; 80: 286-287.

CHAPTER THIRTEEN

PRODUCER INTERESTS IN MEDICINES POLICY

The role of the pharmaceutical industry

Justin Greenwood

INTRODUCTION

A striking feature about the relationships between governments and the pharmaceutical industry in the developed world is their similarities. All governments are concerned with medicine costs, safety, and efficacy. Governments are equally keen to attract and maintain a strong pharmaceutical industry presence as part of their industrial base, not least because it represents one of the world's most successful and profitable types of economic activity. Governments become dependent upon the pharmaceutical industry for their economic contribution, and for the supply of safe and efficacious medicines. In turn, pharmaceutical companies are dependent upon governments as purchasers, as sponsors and as regulators. As a consequence of this power dependence relationship, the supply of medicines to national health care systems typically involves both government and industry in working very closely together on a variety of issues. Sometimes, there are "winners" and "losers"; indeed, the dominance or equality of one partner against the other in this equation is the variable factor between different nations, depending upon the size of the "bargaining chips" possessed by each of the two actors; government and industry, and the degree of organisation of the industry, usually through its trade association.

In Britain, the National Health Service (NHS) is the chief customer of the UK pharmaceutical industry, accounting for 83% of its sales, and representing its sixth largest market in the world. Following oil and advertising, the pharmaceutical industry is the third most profitable industry in the UK. For 40 consecutive years it has contributed to Britain's balance of trade, and in 1990 its contribution surplus amounted to £1 billion, making it the UK's third largest foreign exchange earner from visible trade. Britain has been successful in making itself an attractive base for the pharmaceutical industry to operate from, and consequently it is home to a disproportionately high percentage of world production and research facilities. Three of the five leading prescribed medicines worldwide were discovered in Britain, and the world's best selling prescription medicine, Zantac, has made Glaxo Britain's most successful company. Against a backdrop of national trade deficits, these factors provide highly influential "bargaining chips" which the pharmaceutical industry uses to exert leverage on UK public medicines policy. Two key issues which receive attention here concern the inter-related issues of medicine costs and information provision to prescribers.

THE UK MEDICINES BILL AND THE PHARMACEUTICAL INDUSTRY

In Britain, spending on medicines accounts for 11% (£2.9 billion in 1990[1]) of all NHS expenditure. Since the inception of the NHS in 1948, concerns have continually been expressed about the escalating costs of the national medicines bill. Among the items held responsible are demographic changes, rising health expectations, the increased use of proprietary medicines in prescription writing, the absence of cost consciousness amongst prescribers, the multi-national nature of the pharmaceutical industry, commercial promotional activities and government–industry regulatory relationships. The focus of this chapter is upon these last three items.

In 1957, concerns about escalating medicines costs prompted the Minister of Health to propose a scheme designed to control expenditure. Rather than becoming a victim of government inspired regulation over which it might exert little control, the pharmaceutical industry, through its trade association, the Association of the British Pharmaceutical Industry (ABPI), proposed its co-operation in a price control scheme of its own design. For his part, the Minister of Health, anxious to avoid a confrontation with a key industrial interest with the power to exert influence over the activities of his department, accepted the proposal, resulting in the creation of the "Voluntary Price Regulation Scheme" (VPRS). In 1969, this became the "Pharmaceutical Price Regulation Scheme" (PPRS), inaptly named in that it involved not control over medicine prices, but rather over the profits made by pharmaceutical companies in their trade with the NHS on the basis of companies submitting annual accounts to the Department of Health. Companies with higher levels of investment in the UK were to be permitted higher profit levels in their NHS business, thus making explicit the link between the industry's economic activities and the national medicines bill. The principles of the 1969 PPRS scheme have survived to the present day, and include an agreement between the two parties:

'not only that safe and effective medicines are available on reasonable terms to the National Health Service, but also that a strong, efficient and profitable pharmaceutical industry in the United Kingdom is capable of such sustained research and development expenditure as should lead to the future availability of new and improved medicines, both for the National Health Service and for export'.[2]

This agreement makes explicit the partnership basis on which pharmaceutical policy in the UK is made. The dual, and in some respects conflicting, role of the Department of Health as both sponsor and regulator of the industry, has in part been held responsible by a variety of commentators for the failure of government to control escalating medicines costs.[3] In effect, the "bargaining chips" held by the pharmaceutical industry give it an "inside track" in government – access to key policy making decisions. These "bargaining chips" include government's reliance upon the industry for its contribution to the balance of trade, and upon industry's capacity to provide the NHS with new and improved medicines through its research activities. Industry's ultimate fall back position could be to threaten to take its activities elsewhere. Lindblom argues that:

'whilst government exercises broad authority over business, the exercise of that authority is curbed and shaped by the concern of government officials for its possible adverse effects on business, since adverse effects can cause consequences that government officials are unwilling to accept...the unspoken possibility of adversity for business operates as an all pervasive constraint on government authority'.[4]

Lindblom's argument should not be taken as implying that business interests will win every encounter with government; rather, that business may possess key resources through which it is possible to influence policy making and implementation. Judgments about likely "winners" or "losers" can only be made by studying the cards in the possession of the industry in question. In the case of the pharmaceutical industry, its "aces" make it a particularly strong player. For instance, an apparent "defeat for the pharmaceutical industry",[5] according to Sargent, was the 1977 National Health Service Act, which gave the Minister of Health the power to fix the prices of medicines by order. However, governments have never used these powers, not least because to do so would jeopardise the co-operation of the pharmaceutical industry in price control schemes and other partnership arrangements, and to risk the loss of domestic investment by a highly successful industry. This phenomenon has been called "regulatory capture"[6] – where industry has government in a "Catch 22" situation. Although governments possess the theoretical ability to regulate industry, it is effectively unable to do so. It is for these reasons that the pharmaceutical industry first proposed its involvement in a price control scheme.

One indicator of the success or otherwise of a key interest such as the pharmaceutical industry in achieving its political goals concerns the extent to which it appeals to public opinion for support. In general, the more an interest has to air its demands and grievances in public the less successful it is; often, "going public" indicates that an interest has been unsuccessful in getting its demands met, behind closed doors with government, and it is appealing for public support as a measure of last resort. Using this as an indicator, it is possible to conceive of the relationship between government and the pharmaceutical industry as a settled one, occasionally disrupted by brief periods of turbulence. The pharmaceutical industry made a number of highly publicised threats concerning its future UK investment plans in the period from 1983 to 1985, when it faced a number of serious regulatory issues from government. These included the 1982 Greenfield Report on generic substitution;[7] cuts in profit and promotion levels (1983); and threats of curbs on transfer pricing activities and the limited list of prescribable drugs (1985). Together, these events proved extremely disruptive to the hitherto rather cosy relationship the two parties had enjoyed, and occurred largely as a result of the affairs of the industry coming into the public eye.

The affairs of the pharmaceutical industry reached the public agenda as a result of a number of incidents. One concerned the public hearings (1982-83,[8] 1983-84[9]) of the House of Commons Public Accounts Committee, which concluded that the Department of Health was unable to properly control the prices of medicines under the terms of the PPRS through its lack of resources, and by the nature of its relationship with the industry. Another concerned the cumulative effects of safety crises, most notably the non steroidal anti inflammatory drugs "Opren" and "Flosint". Product licences for these preparations were withdrawn by the Committee on Safety of Medicines (CSM) following their association with serious adverse affects, which in some cases resulted in patient deaths. A series of television documentaries linked these events with the marketing of the products by the two respective manufacturers, involving highly graphic footage of free trips to Venice for prescribers aboard the Orient express, paid for by the companies involved. The unusually high profile of the industry's affairs led to a climate in which regulatory action was inevitable, disrupting the usual partnership approach to medicines' governance whereby the practice had been for issues to be settled behind closed doors, away from the glare of public attention.

The 1982 Greenfield Report on generic substitution represented one of the greatest threats to the industry. The report recommended that pharmacists should have the ability to substitute prescriptions written for branded products with their generic equivalent. The potential savings, projected to be as much as

10% of the national medicines bill, were a matter of considerable alarm to the research-based pharmaceutical industry; Hoechst, for instance, publicly linked the report with its decision to cancel plans for new research laboratories in Milton Keynes. Thus, when government announced its intention not to implement the Greenfield Report, but instead to reduce profit levels and re-imbursable promotional expenditure under the terms of the PPRS, the industry was relatively relieved, not least because of government's inability to accurately assess the levels of these activities. Although there was a simultaneous announcement from the Health Minister to initiate an enquiry into the industry's transfer pricing activities (a complicated set of financial transactions between parent and subsidiary companies in different countries aimed at concealing profit levels in NHS transactions) the enquiry's work was either never concluded or never made public.

However, any view in the industry that it had escaped with minimal damage was to prove short lived, because in 1984 the Health Minister announced his intention to revive an idea first considered by the 1956 Guillebaud Committee of Enquiry into the medicines bill,[10] a "limited list" of drugs available on the NHS. The limited list was proposed for the first time, to restrict the number of drugs in certain therapeutic categories which could be prescribed on the NHS, and, as such, represented a significant threat to the pharmaceutical industry supplying the UK market. The industry, through both the ABPI and individual companies, mounted a high profile public relations campaign aimed at defeating the proposal. The ABPI, for instance, spent £1 million on a newspaper advertising campaign, warning in highly emotive terms that the proposal would result in a two tier NHS whereby patients who were not in a position to do so, would be forced to seek the medicines they needed by private prescription. Similarly, Roche wrote to all general practitioners urging them to bombard members of parliament with contrary opinion. In the event this proved highly counter productive, in that both the ABPI's newly found concern with social justice and its unlikely alliance of opposition with the Labour Party, and the Roche tactics, so incensed Government and some sections of parliamentary opinion that one Conservative MP publicly pledged himself to:

> 'expose the pharmaceutical industry for the self interested money grabbing cartel that it is'.[11]

During the debate over the proposals, the Prime Minister received a delegation of American pharmaceutical executives, one of whom walked off the plane at Heathrow into a press conference to issue dire warnings of the withdrawal of UK investment if the scheme went ahead. By this time, however, the Government had become used to such threats which had in previous years been over employed as a tactic by the industry, and an amended limited list scheme was implemented in 1985 in circumstances of divided opinion amongst both the public and medical professions.

Although the list has not proved the threat to the industry it had at one time imagined, it did demonstrate the capability of government, in certain circumstances, to regulate in cases where it did not see the public interest as co-terminus with those of the pharmaceutical industry. Those circumstances involved the end of a lengthy period during which the affairs of the industry had been very much in the public eye; where its public image had taken a battering from the events of the previous years; and where it had played its "ace card" too often in too short a space of time. The industry found that it could not appeal to a public, as a measure of last resort, whose sympathy for it had been seriously eroded in previous years. These circumstances were unique to the time of the passage of the limited list; the Minister had been able to introduce a scheme against an industry on the defensive with a tarnished reputation. Government's relationship with the pharmaceutical industry since has very much been restored to its previous "behind closed doors" model. Indeed, in the period since 1985 the pharmaceutical industry has enjoyed one of its most settled relationships with government to date, not least because of the withdrawal of public interest after the implementation of the limited list. This enabled government to reverse cuts made to profitably in 1983, largely without public or parliamentary attention. As a consequence, the UK industry has enjoyed one of its most prosperous periods of operation, to the extent that Ministers are again (January 1993) beginning to question whether the public gets value for money from the medicines bill.

The episode of the limited list illustrates the difficulties of working with generalised models of power dependence, in that these are neither static nor universal. In turn, this illustrates the weakness of generalised theories in political science which attempt to characterise the nature of state machinery. Rather, it illustrates a very important concept first suggested by Theodore Lowi in 1964; that "policies make politics", that is that the type of policy under consideration influences the underlying politics.[12] In effect, Lowi is pointing to the futility of making generalisations, particularly across sectors of activities. The uniqueness of each case must be fully appreciated before any judgment can be arrived at; nevertheless, there are a number of useful models available in political science which do help construct images of the relationships between a particular sector of industry and government, rather than attempting to make generalisations about government and industry as a whole. One of these, based on the idea of interest groups, will be used after a discussion of arrangements concerning medicine information.

MEDICINE INFORMATION FOR PRESCRIBERS

Marketing medicines is a crucial activity for pharmaceutical companies. Higgins has argued that:

> 'a pharmaceutical company does not market chemicals, it markets information. Without effective communication there is no transmission of the information, and without the information there is no prescription'.[13]

Governments have been aware for some time that the marketing activities of the pharmaceutical industry inflate the size of the national medicines bill. The 1959 Hinchliffe Committee report into the cost of prescribing,[14] and the 1967 Sainsbury Committee report into the relationship of the government with the pharmaceutical industry[15] were unequivocal. For instance, the Sainsbury Committee Report concluded that:

> 'sales promotion unquestionably plays an important part in inducing doctors to prescribe new products'.[16]

Despite such evidence, it was not until 1976 that a government sought to control the promotional activities of pharmaceutical firms. This involved the introduction of a 14% ceiling on promotional expenditure by pharmaceutical companies (expressed as a proportion of total NHS sales), which, by 1983 had been reduced to 9%, where it presently remains. Not too much should be read into this 5% reduction. Firstly, any pharmaceutical firm may exceed this proportion if it wishes; 9% refers only to expenditure which governments take into account when assessing profit levels under the terms of the PPRS. Secondly, the reductions were easily circumvented. The Department of Health lacks the resources to assess company accounts properly under the PPRS scheme. In addition, companies responded by setting up subsidiary companies, often marketing identical products using two sales forces, who were also entitled to a 9% proportion of promotional activity. Thirdly, the industry could live with any reductions, because the purpose of some of its peripheral marketing activities, such as advertising, was competitive and therefore wasteful; for instance, it enabled firms such as Smith Kline, with cimetidine, and Glaxo, with ranitidine, to cut out 'flag flying' activities such as advertising, and concentrate instead on their more important sales forces, based on the use of medical representatives.

Governments have always allowed the pharmaceutical industry the lion's share in providing information about medicines to prescribers. The pharmaceutical industry spends £50 on this activity for every £1 spent by government, amounting to £5,000 per family doctor per year. Approximately half of this is spent on maintaining sales forces of medical representatives. Around 85 sales forces provide employment for an estimated 4,500+ medical representatives in the UK – around one for every six general practitioners. The industry believes these exert considerable influences upon prescribing behaviour. Alan Sanders, then the Marketing Director of Smith Kline French, told his colleagues at an industry conference:

> 'the Marketing Director knows that adverts and mailings do not sell *per se*. The way the company gets through to the doctor is through its best communicator – the representative. A large percentage of doctors rely on medical representatives for product information, and these doctors at the time of the interview can be influenced'.[17]

A number of studies have demonstrated conclusively the influence of the medical representative upon prescribing behaviour.[18,19,20] In a survey conducted by the author, one general practitioner commented that:

> 'it is usually possible to tell from patients notes which reps called at the practice the previous week'.[21]

Representative effectiveness is achieved through targeting attentions on certain groups of prescribers; typically, a company spends 40-50% of its calling activities on 10-15% of prescribers, these being the highest volume and cost group. A little known fact concerns the ability of the pharmaceutical industry to purchase data which enables it to identify the prescribing practices of doctors. It tends to be the older doctors who are most influenced by representatives – many of whom qualified before the pharmaco-therapeutic revolution, and have become reliant upon the medical representative for updating. To this group, the representative represents a convenient and relatively attractive means of updating. It is the face to face nature of the representative which thus provides the key to their influence, and surveys have found a number of close personal relationships which have developed between representatives and prescribers.[22] In a survey conducted by the author, one general practitioner commented that:

> 'if you like a rep you might give his new product a go'.[23]

Despite government awareness of these influences, and their impact upon both the medicines bill and "rational" prescribing, it prefers to take action more in the field of consumption (patients, doctors, pharmacists) than in that of production (the pharmaceutical industry). In 1988, the Chief Medical Officer at the Department of Health and Social Security (DHSS) told the medical profession:

> 'the responsibility for achieving more effective and economic prescribing now lies with the medical profession. The medical profession must pick up the ball and run with it...we will help, but the move is in your hands'.[24]

Thus, in recent years governments have focused their efforts on controlling costs at groups in the consumption chain of medicine. Doctors now have fund-holding practices; indicative drug budgets; independent medical advisors. Patients are subject to regular rises in prescription charges. Pharmacists are regularly subjected to measures designed to secure all due economy in the nation's medicines bill, and thought of as a vehicle of advice to prescribers. Similarly, governments have been very unwilling to take a proportionately greater role in the provision of information to prescribers, although the advent of the Independent Medical Service does represent a significant innovation for rational prescribing advice. In the main, however, the task of informing doctors is left to the pharmaceutical industry – because this is the key to the industry's prosperity. The point is that governments find it easier and relatively less controversial to take action in consumption fields than it does against powerful economic interests in the production sphere, such as the pharmaceutical industry. This idea is a variation on a theme first discussed by Saunders and Cawson – the "dual state" thesis, whereby state activities in the fields of production and consumption are underpinned by quite different types of politics.[25]

A further illustration of the difficulties the state experiences in acting in certain types of production sectors is provided by the case of the regulation of pharmaceutical marketing. The provision of information to prescribers is formally controlled by the 1968 Medicines Act and its update, the 1972 Medicines (Data Sheet) Regulations. These make it an offence to proffer a false or misleading statement about a medicine, and set out certain conditions under which a medicine may be marketed. However, governments of all shades have preferred not to use the provisions of these instruments, but instead to rely upon self regulation by the pharmaceutical industry. Indeed, only 4 prosecutions have been instigated against individuals for contraventions of the 1968 Medicines Act; and one against a company. In contrast, the Department of Health refers around a dozen cases involving contraventions each year to the self regulatory committee of the ABPI. The view of the Department of Health is officially recorded in an answer to a Parliamentary question; that they defer

> 'to any action taken under the pharmaceutical industry's own self
> regulatory procedures, since these may provide a very effective and speedy
> means of control'.[26]

The ABPI's self regulatory code follows very closely the provisions of the 1968 Medicines Act. Indeed, it has been designed by the industry to do so, precisely because it would prefer to retain control itself over its own marketing activities. La Barbara argues that:

> 'a powerful motivation behind the adoption of self regulation is industry's
> desire to forestall government regulation'.[27]

Thus, each new edition of the code, offering improved provisions, has closely followed the threat of regulation. The first (1957) version followed government's announcement of its intention to regulate, which ultimately resulted in the PPRS; the 1962 update followed the thalidomide crisis; the 1967 series, the Sainsbury Committee report; the 1978 version, the 1977 NHS Act; the 1983 version, the Opren crisis; and the 1986 version, the limited list. The code of practice committee meets to adjudicate upon complaints of transgressions made to it, and dispenses judgments which are in the main reliant upon the deterrent sanction of bad publicity. Until 1983, the committee met and adjudicated in secret, and its sanctions relied mainly upon requests to transgressors not to repeat the offending incident. Thus, the code has been more "window dressing" than a strict attempt at regulation, not least because secret deliberations have failed to warn the medical profession of a problem. One example here again concerns Opren. The manufacturer; Lilly, had indirectly marketed it to the public through press conferences announcing the arrival of a "new breakthrough" in the treatment of arthritis, and the resultant publicity suggested that the drug was effective in moderating the course of the disease rather than relieving the symptoms. Similarly, a promotional video issued to doctors by Lilly underplayed the seriousness of photosensivity reactions. The failure of the ABPI code attracted serious public criticisms, resulting in the release of subsequent findings to public sources – again illustrating the purpose of the code to mainly forestall government regulation.

Self regulatory arrangements can work effectively; that administered by the Advertising Standards Authority, for instance, provides a quick, cheap and efficacious channel of redress for members of the general public; it is also one less thing for governments to have to do, thereby saving time and resources. Self discipline can often work better than restrictive rules, and codes can be interpreted according to the spirit of the law rather than the letter – again assisting the public. Industry also often prefers these arrangements, because it enables them to retain a degree of control over their own affairs. Self regulatory arrangements, as part of a voluntary agreement between government and industry which allows industry to perform the regulatory function in the public interest, can be made to work where the industry believes there is a real regulatory threat posed by government. Speaking of arrangements in the tobacco sector, one time Health Minister Dr David Owen commented that:

'voluntary agreements are not worth the paper they're written on unless the industry concerned knows the Minister has the power to legislate'.[28]

Although governments have theoretically possessed the background legislation necessary to encourage the industry to conduct self regulation properly, in practice the mechanism does not work in full. This is because governments have been reluctant to use their powers under the terms of the 1968 Medicines Act because to do so might jeopardise the involvement of the industry in sectoral governance, including arrangements like the PPRS and the self regulatory code itself. Once again, this illustrates Mitnick's concept of "regulatory capture".

Thus far, it has been possible to employ the concept of power dependence to understand situations in which government and the pharmaceutical industry have become "winners" and "losers" in respect of regulatory events. But the power of the industry operates in several ways. In certain circumstances, it need not even be set in operation to be influential. In others, it needs to be organised by deliberate actions. The remainder of this chapter is devoted to identifying the means through which the pharmaceutical industry exerts influence upon public policy.

THE ABPI AND PUBLIC POLICY

Lindblom's thesis of the privileged position of business in government suggests that key economic interests are automatically influential upon government policy. But if this influence is to be exerted in anything more than a general sense, an interest will need to be organised. The pharmaceutical industry is organised by its trade association, the ABPI. Based in Whitehall premises, only a few hundred yards from key institutions of government, the Association's impressively large secretariat pursues the interests of the industry through its relationship with civil servants, Ministers and MPs, conducted on behalf of its members. Such outlets are generally referred to as "pressure groups", or "interest groups".

Key factors to the success of an interest group include its legitimacy, and the collective "bargaining chips" which it wields on behalf of its members. Legitimacy refers to the recognition given to a group to speak authoritatively on behalf of the interest it represents. Government needs to know that the interest association does represent the bulk of interests in a particular arena, and is therefore able to speak for them. Indeed, governments prefer to deal with industries who have the ability to speak with one collective voice, rather than having to address a plethora of fragmented interests. The ABPI meets this criteria, in that all but two pharmaceutical firms supplying medicines to the NHS are members of it. Governments can thus communicate with the industry when it needs to, by using the ABPI. The "bargaining chips" of the ABPI concern its ability to provide information for government on issues concerning medicines provision on which public policies can be made; the economic contribution of the industry to Britain's balance of trade; and its ability to influence the activities of its members. This latter function occurs through the ability of the ABPI to act as a "one voice" mechanism, enabling it to negotiate with government on behalf of its members; to carry any bargains struck with government over public policies back to its membership; and to ensure that its members "tow the line" in keeping good faith with such deals. An example here concerns the preference of the industry for self regulation. Government allows the industry to self regulate its marketing activities rather than use the provisions of the 1968 Medicines Act, in return for the industry's promise, through the ABPI, to exercise control over its members in agreeing to abide by the self regulatory code. The arrangement keeps both parties happy; the industry retains control over its marketing activities, makes government dependent upon its goodwill, and forestalls further government activities; while for government, there is the advantage that it is spared the expense and time of involvement in detailed affairs of regulation.

These factors, in combination, give the ABPI an "inside track" with government. The influence of groups such as the ABPI is thus far greater than the public and open "pressure groups", whose lack of legitimacy and "bargaining chips" forces them to try to influence government through seeking public attention for the affairs which are claimed to be represented. Having an "inside track" means that an interest enjoys the ability to influence public policies, often away from the glare of public attention, "behind closed doors". The ABPI and government are together locked in a power dependence relationship; governments rely upon the industry for all the factors identified above, while industry relies upon government for promotion and freedom from restrictive legislation. These types of relationships have been characterised by Richardson and Jordan as "policy communities."[29] These are in general settled communities of relationships between the parties involved, often impenetrable to outsiders, and are good mechanisms for resolving disputes and conducting business, contributing to what the same authors characterise as a British "policy making style", based upon the desire to avoid conflict and to settle issues where possible through negotiation and bargaining. Indeed, British government is fragmented into a whole series of "policy communities", involving departments and representatives of the relevant interest, each acting in a "clientilistic" way towards the other. One example concerns the relationship between the Ministry of Agriculture, Fisheries and Food (MAFF) and the National Farmers Union (NFU), a relationship so close that the Ministry is seen as the spokesperson for farming interests inside government. The ABPI and government is another recognisable "policy community". In both of these examples, the communities have evolved into governance mechanisms. The ABPI is very closely involved in the public governance of medicines supply, most notably through its voluntary participation in the PPRS scheme, and through the self regulation of marketing activities. Indeed, the ABPI has in part "crossed the boundary" dividing private interests and those of states, becoming itself part of government by taking on these essentially public functions.

The type of relationship between the ABPI and government in Britain can also be found in other developed countries where the pharmaceutical industry has a strong presence. This is because the issues are essentially the same. Governments like the pharmaceutical industry because of its success, but worry about prices, medicine information and safety. This commonality of experience has enabled the industry to operate cohesively at the European level, where it is organised by the Brussels based European Federation of Pharmaceutical Industry Associations (EFPIA). EFPIA has a very similar relationship with the European Commission as the ABPI does with the UK government. Consequently, it has successfully headed off Commission proposals for the regulation of medicine pricing and information, not least through its ability to enter into power dependence relationships with different parts of the Commission. Thus, EFPIA responded to a threat to regulate its marketing activities by proposing itself as the agency of self regulation for the European industry, proposing a code which is in some instances identical to the British version. In fact, the ability of the industry to work together effectively at the European level has enabled it to achieve far more than was once possible at the national level. For instance, EFPIA persuaded the Commission to take the governments of Italy and Belgium to the European Court of Justice over pricing arrangements which the industries in those countries had once been a party.[30] A similar story can also be told at the global level, where the industry responded to the threat of regulation by the Geneva based World Health Organisation (WHO) by forming the International Federation of Pharmaceutical Manufacturers Associations (IFPMA), located in the same city. Perhaps unsurprisingly, a key strategy used by the IFPMA was in the formation of a self regulatory code of marketing practice in order to assist it in deflecting criticism of its marketing activities.[31]

Pharmacists also have the ability to influence government policies. However, an assessment of the extent to which this is possible would require an analysis of the details of the structure of the sector, its degree of organisation or fragmentation, and the degree to which the "bargaining chips" it holds, such as information, expertise and economic contribution, are key resources sought by different parts of government. Once again, the key concept is power dependence, and once again the methodology of discovery would be through the case study approach advocated by Lowi.[12] These key concepts represent the key contribution which political science can make to understanding the inputs to, processes of, and outputs from, public policies.

REFERENCES

1. Association of the British Pharmaceutical Industry (ABPI) Annual Review. London: ABPI; 1991.
2. Department of Health and Social Security (DHSS) *Pharmaceutical Price Regulation Scheme*. London: DHSS; 1966, p1.

3. For a review of these see Greenwood J. *The Market and the State: the pharmaceutical industry and general medical practice.* Ph.D thesis, University of Nottingham 1988; Chapter 2.

4. Lindblom C. *Politics and Markets.* New York: Basic Books; 1977, p178.

5. Sargent JA. The Politics of the Pharmaceutical Price Regulation Scheme, In: Streeck W, Schmitter PC. *Private Interest Government.* London: Sage; 1985, p121.

6. Mitnick BM. *The Political Economy of Regulation.* New York: Columbia; 1980.

7. Greenfield Report. *Report to the Secretary of State for Social Services of an Informal Working Group on Effective Prescribing.* London: DHSS; 1982.

8. Committee of Public Accounts. *Dispensing of Drugs in the National Health Service.* Tenth report, session 1982-83. London: HMSO; 1983.

9. Committee of Public Accounts. *Dispensing of Drugs in the National Health Service.* Twenty ninth report, session 1983-4. London: HMSO; 1984.

10. Ministry of Health. *Report of the Committee of Enquiry into the Cost of the National Health Service (The Guillebaud Report).* London: HMSO; 1956.

11. Anonymous. MP Launches Attack on the Industry. *The Pharmaceutical Journal* 1985; 234: 6319.

12. Lowi T. American Business, Case Studies, Public Policy and Political Theory. *World Politics* 1964; 16: 677-715.

13. Higgins D. cited in Strickland-Hodge B. *The Impact of Drug Information on the Prescribing of Drugs.* Unpublished Ph.D thesis, University of Aston 1979.

14. Ministry of Health. *Final Report of the Committee on the Cost of Prescribing.* (The Hinchliffe Report) London: HMSO; 1959.

15. Report of the Committee of Enquiry into the Relationship of the Pharmaceutical industry with the National Health Service, 1965-1967 (The Sainsbury Report) London: HMSO; 1969.

16. Ibid. p68.

17. Sanders A. *The New Age of Pharmaceutical Marketing conference.* London: Macfarlane Conferences; 1984, p51.

18. Strickland-Hodge B. *The Impact of Drug Information on the Prescribing of Drugs.* Unpublished Ph.D thesis, University of Aston 1979.

19. Avorn JL. Scientific versus Commercial Sources of Influence upon the Prescribing Behaviour of Physicians. *American Journal of Medicine* 1982; 73: 4-8.

20. Greenwood J. The Market and the State: *The Pharmaceutical Representative and General Medical Practice.* Unpublished Ph.D thesis, University of Nottingham 1988.

21. Ibid. p322.

22. Greenwood J. *Marketing Medicines,* London: Remit; 1988, Chapter 5. Available from Remit Consultants, 422 St John Street, London.

23. Greenwood J. *Marketing Medicines,* London: Remit; 1988, p320.

24. Rational prescribing your responsibility, UK doctors told, *SCRIP* 1985: 1036: 4.

25. Saunders P. *Social Theory and the Urban Question* London: Hutchinson; 1981.

26. HANSARD. Session 1985-86, April 21 – May 2, written answers, 1986: p76.

27. La Barbara P. The Diffusion of Trade Association Advertising Self Regulation. *Journal of Marketing* 1983; 47: 58.

28.Taylor P. *The Smoke Ring: Tobacco, Money and International Politics.* London: Spherem; 1984, p87.
29.Richardson JJ, Jordan AG. *Governing Under Pressure.* Oxford: Martin Robertson; 1979.
30.Greenwood J, Ronit K. Pharmaceutical Regulation in Denmark and the UK: reformulating interest representation to the transnational level. *European Journal of Political Research* 1991; 19: 327-359.
31.Greenwood J. The Regulation of Pharmaceutical Marketing by National Governments; Towards a Transnational Private Interest Government? conference paper, joint sessions, European Consortium for Political Research: Paris: 1989.

CHAPTER FOURTEEN

WHAT DO HOSPITAL PHARMACISTS DO ON THE WARDS?

Nick Barber, Ros Batty and Elizabeth Beech

INTRODUCTION

By the 1960's drug therapy within hospitals had become complex as an ever increasing range of drugs were available. It became evident that the existing systems which had been used to order and supply drugs to the ward would no longer be able to cope. Research carried out in the USA[1] and in Britain[2,3] found that on occasions patients were either receiving the wrong drugs or doses, or not even receiving drugs at all. These countries adopted different solutions: in the USA a pharmacist would prepare the doses for each patient each day – this is called unit dose; in Britain the solution was a team approach which involved a new system of prescribing and supplying drugs within hospitals.

The team approach centred round a unique pro-forma prescription sheet which was to stay with the patient at all times, usually at the foot of the bed. The ward would keep commonly used drugs as stock, and a pharmacist would visit the ward daily to check whether the patient had been prescribed any drugs that were not stocked on the ward and, if this was found to be the case, they would initiate a supply of the drug specifically for that patient. This was the first time that hospital pharmacists had ventured outside of the confines of the pharmacy and meant that they saw in-patients for the first time and were able to see how they received their medication. It also meant that pharmacists became part of the ward team. Communication between health care workers was improved and the pharmacist was permitted to make a more significant contribution to therapy. The benefits were quickly recognised and the system, called "ward pharmacy", became recommended practice.[4,5]

The system of ward pharmacy in itself has developed little during the last 25 years. There has, however, been a change in relation to the pharmacist's role, which has been extended in terms of assessing the suitability of drug therapy for the patient. The individualising of drug therapy for each patient, which can take place both on and off the ward, has become known as "clinical pharmacy". It has been supported both by the independent Nuffield Inquiry[6] and by the Government[7] and now most schools of pharmacy offer postgraduate qualifications in clinical pharmacy. Despite these developments, there has as yet been little work in the UK (and little work of good quality anywhere in the world) evaluating the effectiveness of clinical pharmacy or exploring the clinical role that pharmacists play on the ward.

In 1989 a Government White Paper changed the face of the National Health Service (NHS), creating opportunities and threats for clinical pharmacy. The reforms to the NHS were stimulated by reports that the NHS was effective, but not necessarily efficient, and that competition would improve efficiency and shift resources to the better sites. Under the new system there would be a number of health purchasers around the country who would tender for the health care they needed. Hospitals would provide the health care and compete with each other for contracts, which would go to the lowest bidder. To ensure that driving down costs did not compromise quality there would be at least two quality assurance mechanisms. The first was that the purchaser would specify certain quality criteria in their contract, the second was the encouragement of medical audit.

A further important change was the decentralisation and professionalisation of decision making from the hospital manager to directorates, usually headed by a clinician supported by a nurse and a manager. These directorates took care of management and budgets for a section such as "medicine" or "haematology". The control of budgets brought power, and allowed the director to trade off medical against nursing staff or nurses against equipment in order to increase efficiency. One of the budgets they generally took over was their own drug budget, previously managed by the pharmacy department. Moreover, the director, in some hospitals, could choose the nature and extent of the pharmacy service purchased.

The threats to pharmacy that resulted from the new form of the NHS were that manpower (the largest source of expenditure) would be reduced and that it would lose the ability to determine the level of service to each ward. The opportunities came from the quality methods – first, pharmacy needed to convince purchasers that a clinical pharmacy service should be part of each purchasing contract; second, it needed to establish its clinical expertise and have it recognised as part of the medical audit process.

As Regional Health Authority specialists in clinical pharmacy we were concerned that it would be impossible to define the quality of an unmeasured service such as clinical pharmacy and that the downward pressure on staff costs would result in it being attenuated until pharmacy reverted to a supply and compounding service. We therefore decided to measure the nature and extent of current clinical pharmacy activities in ward pharmacy. This was done in the two studies presented here, conducted in and for North West Thames Regional Health Authority. The first constitutes a work sampling study to establish how pharmacists spend their time on the wards and, in particular, the balance between their clinical and supply roles. The second goes on to examine the major part of the clinical role – prescription monitoring and the resulting clinical interventions made by pharmacists. The relationship between their clinical role and the pharmacists' overall workload is also explored. The two studies will be outlined in turn and then their implications will be discussed in more general terms, particularly how they can be used to improve effectiveness and efficiency.

1: WORK SAMPLING STUDY

This study addresses the simple question: What tasks do pharmacists do on wards? To this end a self-reporting multi-dimensional work sampling measure was devised. Work sampling involves the recording of a large number of samples of a worker's tasks using defined and mutually exclusive criteria[8]. Here we describe the development and application of such a measure, and discuss its potential application in the evaluation of pharmacy practice.

Method

Mutually exclusive criteria were developed for two dimensions of work, which were labelled "activity" and "contact". The criteria were discussed with the study pharmacists, piloted for three days, discussed again and then refined. Definitions and examples were provided for each criterion (Figure 1). Six pharmacists providing a twice daily ward pharmacy service to six acute wards recorded their work over five consecutive days. Each visit was classified as a "full visit" if all patients' prescription sheets were checked, or a "walk on, walk off" visit if the pharmacist just checked whether any work was required. An electronic bleeper that emits an audible signal at a random preset frequency was used to prompt pharmacists to record their work. The activity and contact criteria were printed as both text and bar codes on a sheet of paper for use with the ward pharmacy folder. Using a small bar code reader (Figure 2), pharmacists scanned one "activity" criterion followed by one "contact" criterion. The bar code reader automatically dated and timed each scan sequence, and pharmacists also scanned "leave" and "return" bar codes on leaving and returning to the department. For each dimension the number of records for each criterion was expressed as a proportion of the total number of samples (±95% confidence intervals).

DIMENSION	CRITERIA	DESCRIPTION
ACTIVITY	Prescription monitoring	Checking the prescription chart and monitoring for safety, efficacy and economy, including the identification of prescription monitoring incidents. This includes inpatient and TTA prescriptions
	Prescription annotation	Annotation of the prescription with administration details, generic/approved name, dose and/or strength. This does not include supply details
	Information gathering	The gathering of information related to drug therapy and/or patient monitoring
	Change in drug treatment/patient monitoring	Action or attempted action taken to cause a change in drug treatment or patient monitoring
	Stock control	This includes all activity, advice and information relating to the supply, storage and destruction of medicines
	Advice/information	The provision of advice and / or information on any topic with the exception of stock control and change in drug treatment/patient monitoring
	Travel	This includes travel between the pharmacy and one or more wards, and travel between wards, This does not include travel whilst on the ward
	Waste/wait	Time wasted, or spent waiting on the ward
	Personal/Public relations	This includes personal rest time, coffee breaks, social activities, also chat with patients
	Other	Any activity not described in the above categories
CONTACT	Self	The pharmacist participating in the study is the only contact
	Patient	The pharmacist is communicating with the patient
	Pharmacy	The pharmacist is communicating with other pharmacy staff
	Doctor	The pharmacist is communicating with a member of the medical staff, including students
	Nurse	The pharmacist is communicating with a member of the nursing staff, including students
	Other	Individuals not listed in the above definitions

Figure 1: Criteria and definition of work sampling dimensions

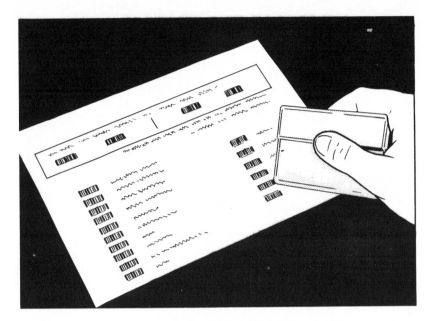

Figure 2: Line drawing of bar codes and time wand

Results

The six ward pharmacists recorded data for 51 ward visits (29 "full visits", 22 "walk-on, walk off" visits). The total time spent on ward visits was 26 hours and 57 minutes; the median time spent on a full visit was 41 minutes, and on a walk-on visit 12 minutes. A total of 417 work measurement samples were recorded, of which one incorrectly scanned record has been excluded. The proportion of records for both "activity" and "contact" criteria are shown in Table 1.

Ward pharmacists spent approximately half their time on clinical pharmacy activities, and a sixth of their time on supply related tasks. For 41% of the time pharmacists were in contact with other people. Of the time spent with patients approximately half involved information gathering, and a third providing advice/information. Ward pharmacists found the bar code reader quick, easy and fun to use. Each bar code reader took about 90 seconds to down load data at the end of each day.

Discussion

Multi-dimensional work sampling can identify what work pharmacists do on the wards. The results show ward pharmacists spent $31.2 \pm 4.4\%$ ($\pm 95\%$ confidence intervals) of their time prescription monitoring and information gathering. This

TABLE 1: Activity and contact

ACTIVITY		CONTACT	
Percent occurrence ± 95% confidence intervals (n=416)		**Percent occurrence ± 95% confidence intervals (n=416)**	
Prescription monitoring	14.5 ± 3.4	Self	59.1 ± 4.7
Prescription annotation	4.3 ± 1.9	Patient	10.3 ± 2.9
Information gathering	16.8 ± 3.6	Pharmacy	3.6 ± 1.8
Change in drug treatment/patient monitoring	4.8 ± 2.0	Doctor	9.4 ± 2.8
Provision of advice/information	8.5 ± 2.7	Nurse	13.7 ± 3.3
Stock control	16.6 ± 3.6	Other	3.9 ± 1.9
Travel	14.2 ± 3.3		
Waste/wait	5.3 ± 2.1		
Personal/Public Relations	6.3 ± 2.3		
Other	8.7 ± 2.7		

result is similar to that obtained in a previous observation of ward pharmacists' activities in a London teaching hospital[9]. Pharmacists spent 6.3 ± 2.3% of their time on personal/public relation activities. The ward pharmacist is frequently the only member of the pharmacy department that ward-based staff meet on a daily basis, and is usually the only member of the pharmacy department seeing in-patients during their hospital stay. Therefore the ward pharmacist's public relations role, while usually undefined, is a small but valuable component of the ward pharmacy service. Pharmacists spent 14.2 ± 3.3% of their time travelling between wards and the pharmacy department; they currently need to return to the pharmacy department to deliver drug supply requests to the dispensary and to return to other duties. The use of electronic data transmission systems and/or full time ward pharmacists could reduce time spent travelling and allow more efficient use of the pharmacists time.

The novel use of technology made data collection fast, easy and direct, removing the possibility of errors associated with indirect data entry. Self-reporting by ward pharmacists had the advantage of avoiding incorrect classification of cognitive tasks by an observer, and of allowing many pharmacists to be studied simultaneously without the need for additional researchers. Accuracy of the work sampling measure was promoted by involving ward pharmacists in the development of the dimension criteria, by the provision of training, and by the daily review of data by the researcher.

This work measure can be used to evaluate the efficiency of different models of ward pharmacy such as once versus twice daily visits. In a wider context it has many applications in both hospital and community practice. For example, it could be used to audit current practice, to identify training needs and for the evaluation of new work practices and technologies in the delivery of pharmaceutical care.

2: PRESCRIPTION MONITORING STUDY

An annual prescription monitoring survey was first set up by two of the authors (N.Barber and R.Batty) in North West Thames Regional Health Authority in 1990. It was designed to study the following:

i. the nature and extent of pharmacists' activity as a consequence of monitoring prescriptions
ii. the time taken to perform ward pharmacy services across the Region
iii. the relationship between ward pharmacist workload and an indicator of their prescription monitoring activity on the wards.

This would allow quantification of one of the pharmacists' contributions to patient care, and would also allow investigation of workers' relative efficiency, allowing comparison between sites.

Method

All 31 acute hospitals in the North West Thames Regional Health Authority which had pharmacies on site were included in the survey. Over a 7 day period in June 1990, June 1991 and June 1992 all pharmacists who visited wards recorded details of the ward they visited, the number of beds on the ward, its speciality, the frequency of ward pharmacy visits, the time they entered and left each ward, the number of endorsements made to clarify administration instructions on prescription sheets and the number of prescription monitoring events (PMEs) that occurred. A PME was defined as any event, usually triggered by reading the prescription, which caused the pharmacist to doubt the appropriateness of a prescription and to take further action to ensure that the prescription was appropriate. Pharmacy staff recorded where the PMEs were identified and by whom, the nature of the event, and the outcome of the PME. The 1990 survey data has been reported in detail elsewhere[10,11].

Results and Discussion

All NHS hospitals in the Region participated in the study. Table 2 shows that over a three year period there was an increase in the number of acute wards and beds visited by pharmacists, the number of PMEs encountered and in the number of ward pharmacists visiting the wards.

TABLE 2: Number of wards, beds etc

	31 Acute Hospitals			40 Non-Acute Hospitals
	1990	1991	1992	1992
No. WARDS	489	497	525	195
No. BEDS VISITED	10337	10592	10871	3807
No. WARD PHARMACISTS	210	226	248	45
No. PMEs	3273	3939	4597	380
No. PMEs/100 BEDS/WEEK	32	37	42	10

The nature of the PMEs (Table 3) were fairly consistent over time and even between acute and non-acute hospitals. For the acute units the events involving dose or frequency, choice of treatment, and administration or formulation or route were consistently the highest. In the non-acute units these events were first, third and fourth respectively, with illegal, illegible or incomplete prescriptions being a more frequent occurrence in the non-acute units than the acute units. Not surprisingly problems related to discharge prescriptions were identified much less frequently in the non-acute units than in the acute units.

The most common outcome for PMEs identified in all years was "prescription altered" (Table 4). When pharmacists offered drug related advice to prescribers, it was rejected in only 4% (1990), 3% (1991) and 3% (1992) of cases in the acute units and in only 2% of cases in the non-acute units.

A performance indicator was derived to encourage comparison between hospitals and identification of good practice; this was PMEs per 100 beds per week (Table 2). For the acute hospitals it ranged from 4 to 82 (median 30) in 1990, from 2 to 123 (median 35) in 1991 and from 4 to 156 (median 39) in 1992. When split by speciality the greatest number of PMEs per 100 beds per week were in intensive therapy units. Work study data also allowed the calculation of

TABLE 3: Nature of PMEs per 100 beds visited at least once in a 7 day period

	Acute Hospitals						Non-Acute Hospitals	
	1990		1991		1992		1992	
Nature of event	No./100 beds	rank	No./100 beds	rank	No./100 beds	rank	No./100 beds	rank
Dose or frequency	9.0	1	10.8	1	12.7	1	2.4	1
Choice of treatment	4.5	2	6.7	2	7.8	2	1.5	2
Administration or formulation or route	4.3	3	5.0	3	6.2	3	1.3	4
Discharge prescription problem	3.3	4	3.2	5	3.8	6	0.3	11=
Prescription illegal or illegible or incomplete	2.8	5	3.1	6	4.0	5	1.9	2
Duration	2.2	6	2.3	9	3.3	7	1.0	5=
Formulary or blacklist	2.1	7=	2.8	7	2.8	8	0.9	7=
Therapeutic drug level monitoring and pharmacokinetics	2.1	7=	2.4	8	2.5	9	1.0	5=
Adverse drug reactions	2.1	7=	3.7	4	5.1	4	0.9	7=
Interaction or incompatibility	1.5	11	1.8	10	1.7	10=	0.3	11=
Pharmacology	0.5	12	0.5	12	0.5	12	0.4	10
Miscellaneous	1.7	10	1.2	11	1.7	10=	0.6	9
Not stated	0.1	13	0	13	0	13	0	13

TABLE 4: Reported outcome for PMEs identified

	Acute Hospitals						Non-Acute Hospitals	
	1990		1991		1992		1992	
Outcome	No.	%	No.	%	No.	%	No.	%
Prescription altered	1611	49	1938	49	2530	55	162	43
Information only	580	18	595	15	552	12	63	17
Incident resolved without intervention	443	14	500	13	594	13	43	11
Prescription unchanged, advice accepted	403	12	608	15	624	14	61	16
Prescription unchanged, advice not accepted	81	3	73	2	88	2	4	1
Not specified	132	4	104	3	102	2	15	4
Unresolved by end of study	23	<1	121	3	107	2	32	8
Total	3273		3939		4597		380	

a second performance indicator – the time to review 100 prescriptions, calculated within each speciality to allow better comparability.

Over the 3 years of the study, these two performance indicators have been developed by sub-dividing them to take into account the fact that some pharmacists monitor prescription sheets at the foot of the patients' beds while others review the sheets at a central point on the ward. This also allows testing of the hypothesis that the two methods of reviewing the prescription are equally effective. The 1992 performance indicator data for the 5 most common specialities are shown in Table 5. The general trend is that when the prescription sheets are located centrally, the pharmacists take less time to look at them and fewer PMEs are generated, supporting the contention that additional information is gained by seeing the patient, as well as their prescription sheet.[12] Pharmacy managers have found these performance indicators useful, allowing them to compare themselves with the Regional mean and to look at differences

TABLE 5: Effect of the location of prescription sheets on the PMEs/100 beds/week and on time to monitor 100 prescription sheets/week. Taken for the 5 most common specialities in acute units in 1992

Speciality	Location of prescription sheets	Median (range) PMEs/100 beds/week	Median (range) Time/100 prescription sheets (hr:min)	No of hospitals
Intensive therapy units	at central point	42 (0–100)	6:56 (3:33 – 20:00)	8
	end of patients' beds	100 (20 – 614)	9:44 (5:39 – 22:37)	22[1]
Medicine	at central point	38 (10 – 43)	2:40 (2:07 – 4:02)	6
	end of patients' beds	46 (8 – 121)	3:20 (1:52 – 4:55)	23[2]
Geriatrics	at central point	17 (0 – 60)	1:44 (0:50 – 4:54)	11
	end of patients' beds	34 (9 – 73)	2:48 (1:26 – 4:25)	18
Surgery	at central point	14 (5 – 15)	2:58 (1:48 – 4:33)	7
	end of patients' beds	25 (5 – 107)	3:03 (1:29 – 4:14)	26[3]
Paediatrics	at central point	13 (0 – 129)	3:32 (2:16 – 7:07)	11[4]
	end of patients' beds	23 (0 – 118)	3:40 (2:15 – 18:20)	21[5]

Notes:
1. n = 21 for data on time to monitor 100 prescription sheets
2. n = 21 for data on time to monitor 100 prescription sheets
3. n = 24 for data on time to monitor 100 prescription sheets
4. n = 10 for data on time to monitor 100 prescription sheets
5. n = 19 for data on time to monitor 100 prescription sheets

between pharmacists covering the same ward specialities. The fact that managers found the study useful probably resulted in improved data collection (and possibly "intervention hunting") and may partly account for the increase in interventions each year.

The survey in the non-acute units was conducted as a pilot to obtain a "snapshot" of pharmacists' inpatient prescription monitoring activities in long stay facilities. The results are shown in Tables 2–4, set against the findings for acute units. In the one week study, 3807 (57%) of the 6656 non-acute beds in the Region were visited at least once, and 8% of the PMEs identified were unresolved at the end of the survey. In terms of number of PMEs per 100 beds per week the non-acute hospitals were consistently lower than the acute hospitals. We will be having discussions with the non-acute unit pharmacy managers to enable us to explore these differences.

IMPLICATIONS OF THESE STUDIES

We started with a simple aim – that of measuring the extent and nature of pharmacists' clinical activities on wards. It is worth examining the fact that we not only achieved this, but found new insights into the nature of pharmacy and in ways of quality assuring it.

The work presented in this chapter shows that clinical pharmacy is a substantial part of a ward pharmacist's role, both from the point of view of time they spend and the changes to therapy that result. The amount of time pharmacists spend talking to staff and patients shows that they interact with others on the ward. The extent of pharmacists' interventions on therapy was much greater than might have been expected. Examination of the individual records has led us to move away from the PMEs – the main indicator, as there seems to be some difference in its interpretation between sites. We now use the more definitive 'number of prescriptions changed' as a marker. In 1992 there was the equivalent (a stay of one week assumed) of one in four prescriptions changed in acute units following advice from a pharmacist.

The nature of the PMEs was the next insight. There is a school of thought, prominent among some members of the medical profession, which admits that pharmacists get prescriptions changed, but assumes that it is on bureaucratic matters such as enforcing formularies or incorrect writing up of controlled drugs. A view held by some pharmacists is that their major role is to pick up interactions, adverse drug reactions and make pharmacokinetic interventions. Our findings suggest that neither one of these speculations is correct. The majority of PMEs that pharmacists identify are to do with the fundamentals of prescribing – giving the right drug in the right dose, form and frequency. In other words, we seem to be carrying out an audit on prescribing, and the clinicians feel pharmacists' advice worth acting on. This has lead us to propose a new role for pharmacy as a routine part of medical audit,[10,13] an activity promoted as part of the changes to the NHS. Involvement in medical audit has been pursued by a few individual pharmacies[14,15] and is an area in which we are still conducting research; it provides a new "value added" role for pharmacy and may help preserve ward pharmacy.

The third important finding comes from standardising our data and then comparing it between sites. Standardisation according to the number of occupied beds or prescription sheets allows some comparison to be made between the sites. Differences may reflect a number of factors such as the "case mix" of the hospital or the quality of its doctors, but may also reflect on the ability of the pharmacists and the systems of work. In similar sites it would be a marker of the clinical pharmacy service to the ward. It is likely that for District General Hospitals, for example, the case mix will be fairly similar, as will the quality of the prescribers. The large range of PMEs /100 beds/week suggests marked differences in the performance of the pharmacists, and we need to find out why they exist. The data is now being modelled using Poisson regression to determine the relationship between high rates of changes to prescriptions and factors such as, education, year of registration,or time spent on the wards. In the

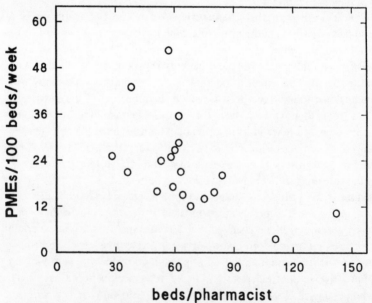

Figure 3: Relationship between beds/ward pharmacist and number of PMEs/100 beds/week for 19 district general hospitals.
Spearmans $r_s = -0.65$, $r^2 = 38.7\%$, p = 0.003

future we will also be investigating the attitudes of ward pharmacists as this may be another major factor influencing their performance. Preliminary analysis shows that one of the factors may be workload. Figure 3 demonstrates that there is an inverse relationship between the number of PME's and the number of beds pharmacists have to visit. One explanation of this relationship would be that the pharmacists with a large number of beds to cover, spend less time looking for or acting on prescriptions of a questionable standard. Further work is being undertaken to determine whether this is a causal relationship.

These measures will allow us to compare different systems of pharmacy in Britain and internationally. They are also a first attempt at deriving measures of efficiency and effectiveness and justifying the role of clinical pharmacy in the NHS. Having access to this data allows pharmacy managers to see their own service in comparison to others in a way not previously available. For example, they can see how long their staff take to cover medical wards in comparison to those in a similar hospital. What is more, the Regional Health Authority, who oversee the work carried out within hospitals, will be able to monitor activity. Regional clinical pharmacy staff in North West Thames visit each site every two years to help develop clinical pharmacy services, using the data we have derived to help identify sub-optimal systems or levels of staff performance. Three case studies can be used to illustrate this.

In hospital A the percentage of PMEs relating to discharge prescriptions was lower in 1990 and in 1991 (5% and 3% respectively) than the Regional means (11% and 8% respectively). The possible reasons for these discrepancies were:

i.   low bed turnover
ii. accurate discharge prescribing by clinicians
iii. no pharmacy system for checking discharge prescriptions prior to dispensing.

Examination of hospital records indicated that reason (i) was not the case. It was thought that both reasons (ii) and (iii) were possible. Procedures for dealing with discharge prescription by pharmacists were revised. The effectiveness of these measures is shown by the results for 1992: the percentage of PMEs was 12% for hospital A compared to a Regional mean of 9%.

At hospital B the ward pharmacists aimed to see not less than 90% of prescriptions on all medical wards. In 1991 the percentage of prescriptions seen for medical ward x, y and z were 96%, 100% and 86% respectively and thus the standard was not being met for ward z. Possible reasons for this included:

i.   inefficient or lazy ward pharmacist
ii. nurses were sending the prescription sheets to the pharmacy department rather than leaving them on the ward for the pharmacist to monitor

iii.   a high number of patients were off the ward at the time of the pharmacist's visit e.g. having endoscopies

iv.   the pharmacist for ward z needed further training.

Further investigation showed that in general a high proportion of patients were off the ward at the time of the pharmacist's ward visit and a decision was made to change the time of the pharmacist's visits to ward z.

The final example occurred at hospital C where there were three similar medical wards l, m and n. The PMEs/100 beds for wards l, m and n were 76, 69 and 50, and the times to review 100 prescriptions for these wards were 3¼ h, 3½ h and 7½ h respectively. Thus ward n took the longest to cover and yet generated the fewest PMEs. Possible reasons for this were:

i.   case mix

ii.   differences between clinicians

iii.   differences between pharmacists.

The case mix was found to be similar and no obvious differences between the clinicians on the three wards could be found. However, ward l and m were covered by the same pharmacist, while ward n was covered by a different pharmacist who gave the impression to her manager of being slow and methodical. It was decided that the pharmacist visiting ward n would receive accompanied visits and further training.

On the basis of the research reported here, the authors can advise on ways of making the system as efficient and effective as possible even against a background of a cut in resources; it may be possible to show the detrimental effect of reductions in the clinical component of service if services are cut too far. The annual prescription monitoring survey has thus led to the development of a quality assurance service for clinical pharmacy.

We have recently been involved in agreeing with other groups of researchers a standardised way of collecting data[16] to allow easier comparison between sites. The clinical importance of the interventions also needs to be assessed using a multidisciplinary approach; which in turn leads to research into the appropriateness of prescribing. We also need to evaluate other clinical pharmacy influences on prescribing which may affect the clinical activity in ward pharmacy; an example would be the measurement of the pharmacist's contribution to consultant ward rounds. As these tools are developed we will be able to evaluate different models of service delivery, including automation and the use of expert systems. Our findings should help purchasing health authorities to set quality standards for ward pharmacy services and help managers of good quality pharmacies justify their services to directorates.

REFERENCES

1. Barker KN, McConnell WE. Detecting errors in hospitals. *American Journal of Hospital Pharmacy* 1962; 19: 360-369.
2. Vere DW. Errors of complex prescribing. *The Lancet* 1965; i: 370-373
3. Crooks J, Clark CG. Prescribing and administration of drugs in hospital. *The Lancet* 1965; i: 373-378.
4. DHSS. Measures for controlling drugs on the wards. *Report of the joint subcommittee on measures for controlling drugs on the wards.* London, HM[70]36, 1970.
5. DHSS. *Report of the working party on the hospital pharmaceutical service.* London, HMSO, 1970.
6. Nuffield Committee of Inquiry into Pharmacy. *Pharmacy: A report to the Nuffield Foundation.* London: The Nuffield Foundation; 1986.
7. Department of Health. *Health services management. The way forward for hospital pharmaceutical services.* London: Department of Health; 1988; HC[88]54.
8. Rascati KL, Kimberlin CL, McCormick WC. Work measurement in pharmacy research. *American Journal of Hospital Pharmacy* 1986; 43: 2445-2452.
9. Jenkins D, Cairns C, Barber N. How do ward pharmacists spend their time?: An activity sampling study. *International Journal of Pharmacy Practice* 1992; 1: 148-151.
10. Batty R, Barber ND. Ward pharmacy: a foundation for prescribing audit? *Quality in Health Care* 1992; 1: 5-9.
11. Barber ND, Blackett A, Batty R. Does a high ward pharmacist's workload decrease their clinical monitoring? *International Journal of Pharmacy Practice* 1993; 2: 152-155.
12. Batty R, Barber ND. Prescription monitoring for ward pharmacists. *The Pharmaceutical Journal* 1991; 247: 242-244.
13. Barber N. Improving quality of drug use through hospital directorates. *Quality in Health Care* 1993; 2: 3-4.
14. Davies G. Clinical audit – a new development. *The Pharmaceutical Journal* 1989; HS30-HS31.
15. Barber N, Eccles S, Frater A, Wilson P. A better pill to swallow. *Health Service Journal* 1992; 102: 22-23.
16. Barber ND, Batty R, Cousins D, Fahey M and Wind K. Minimum data set for hospital prescription monitoring event packages. *The Pharmaceutical Journal* 1992; 249: 346.

CHAPTER FIFTEEN

TEACHING AND LEARNING IN PHARMACY

Ian Bates, David Webb and Janie Sheridan

INTRODUCTION

Pharmacists have until recently been trained to perform essentially manipulative tasks. However, pharmacy is becoming a more complex, problem-solving discipline which draws on not only the natural, but also the behavioural and social sciences. The undergraduate education process is one key to pharmacy's continued evolution and development. Schools of pharmacy however, have traditionally reacted slowly, providing little incentive for course design exercises or even lacking the educational skills required for curriculum design. The development of undergraduate curricula is an appropriate method to enhance professional behaviour and attitudes. Indeed without such developments there can be no advancement of the vocational degree. Commensurately, without a change in graduate behaviour, new professional roles cannot be fully realised.

Education is about equipping individuals with knowledge and skills, and the primary concern must always be to equip undergraduates for the future goals of the profession. This often requires modification of prevailing attitudes and beliefs about the nature of the educational process. This chapter will indicate ways in which the educational process can facilitate change if applied properly, and why it can be a powerful tool for the development of the profession. To understand more about these processes, some insight into the theories surrounding the learning process is necessary.

THEORIES OF LEARNING

Equipped with an understanding of the theories of learning, it should be possible for teachers to apply learning psychology to "everyday" teaching situations. Moreover, curriculum change and curriculum design are necessary in order to underpin and change the profession "bottom up". This can only rationally take place when the precepts of learning psychology drive new teaching methods. Over the course of this century, three main strands of learning theories have evolved. The foremost are the behaviouristic and the cognitive groups, whilst the third group comprises a blend of social and personality psychological theories.

Behaviourist Theories

The behaviourist group formulated the "stimulus-response" or S-R theories of learning, and had an essentially mechanistic approach to the psychology of learning. These theories are concerned primarily with the mechanisms of responses to stimuli. The early works of Skinner, for example, illustrated the principle of operant conditioning, whereby animals were rewarded with food for exhibiting a type of behaviour.[1] A rat randomly running around a cage may accidentally activate a lever, which in turn presents a food pellet to the animal. Learned behaviour stems from the fact that the rat may then repeatedly activate this lever for a food reward. Reinforcement of this particular lever-pressing behaviour may lead to variations and discrimination by the animal; for instance, selecting a particular lever to press. The animals may be rewarded (have their behaviour reinforced) sequentially, leading to quite complex learned behaviour patterns.

In the human context, the key assumption of operant conditioning is that a person's behaviour is directly affected by the consequences of that behaviour. Blackman[2] terms this process the A-B-C of conditioning ('A' is the antecedent conditions, 'B' is the behaviour, 'C' are the consequences). In the context of teaching and learning, general reinforcers will augment a range of different responses. This may include positive feedback from teachers ("good...well done", etc.), feelings of self-esteem and the esteem of colleagues, or material benefits (money for instance). Reinforcers need not be regular, or indeed consistent. Often irregular reinforcers are more powerful in terms of changing behaviour. It is also evident that in order to change a set of behaviours, the teacher should be able to assess how the present reinforcers are acting; in other words how is present behaviour attributable and how will other reinforcers modify that behaviour. If, for example, student attendance for a class or lectures is low, how can a reduction of the reinforcement leading to this behaviour be achieved and how can the classes be changed to reinforce class attendance by the student population?

The Cognitive Theories

Cognitive theorists rejected the purely mechanistic approach of behaviourists. A cognitive approach, for example, would maintain that learners are not simply responding to stimuli in a passive manner, but instead select the important parts of the stimulus, encoding and processing it, and respond in a selective manner depending on prevailing circumstances. The meaning of the stimulus itself is important. In the context of the teaching process, cognitive theorists stress the importance of prior knowledge in relation to new learning. In assessing learners' prior experience, the teacher makes a valuable contribution by helping them select and perceive information. A past experience or interpretation of past events, may engender a "mind set", which can be useful (by facilitating responses) or unhelpful, perhaps by hindering an objective reaction. Teachers need to recognise and correct unhelpful mind sets in order to develop effective learning methods.

The cognitive approach has also facilitated the idea of "latent learning" such that a segment of learning could take place which would not become apparent in behaviour until some later date. Teachers should be able to introduce ideas at an early stage which will aid the development of more difficult concepts at a later stage. One other important development of the cognitive approach suggests that people are able to rearrange existing knowledge and cognitive skills in order to solve new problems. The design of the curriculum and teachers should facilitate this process, using appropriate teaching strategies and methods as tools.

Social and Personality Psychology and Motivation

Clearly individuals will learn more effectively if they are motivated to do so. It is less obvious what the precise nature of motivation is, or how it can be assessed and encouraged. Herzberg[3] argues that motivational factors fall into two groups, both of which affect feelings of self esteem, but in opposite ways. High esteem tends to be associated with the learning experience itself, particularly a task or problem-based experience. Learners like to be able to complete exercises, and feel good about themselves when this happens, particularly when coupled with acknowledgements of completion. A sense of responsibility grows and individuals feel more able to take responsibility for their own learning. Conversely, feelings of low esteem are associated with deficiencies within the learning environment. These may include poor teaching, feelings of low status in the peer and tutor group, or poor teaching environments and result in feelings of unfairness and an unsatisfactory outlook among students. However, it is suggested that these environmental factors may not be of equal importance and that improving the immediate environment may ameliorate feelings of dissatisfaction, but not completely reverse them. It is much more important to improve the learning experiences and tasks, making them more meaningful for learners. This results in a marked improvement in satisfaction and self-esteem.

Additionally, the self-esteem of learners is affected by the attitudes of teachers, and the judgement of the latter concerning the motivation of the former often governs the selection of teaching methods. The way in which students view their teachers will similarly affect motivation. It is possible to construct a spectrum of teachers' attitudes and examine the opposing poles of this continuum. On the one hand, a general teaching strategy held by a teacher may be that students are inherently work-shy, disliking work to the extent of avoiding it if at all possible. The other extreme contends that students enjoy mental effort just as much as physical effort associated with "play" and recreation.

Within the framework of the three main categories of learning theory, Hilgard and Bower[4] describe a series of principles which could be applied to the practice of teaching (Table 1).

TABLE 1

Application of Learning Theory in Practice

Themes relating to Behaviourism:
Activity
Repetition
Reinforcement

Themes relating to Cognitive Approaches
Understanding
Organisation and Structure
Perception
Cognitive Feedback
Interpersonal Differences

Themes relating to Social and Personal Psychology
Learning as a Natural Process
Purpose
Social Environment
Anxiety and Emotions
Responsibility and Relevance.

Adapted from reference 4

Taking the three main groups of themes by turn, it is argued that learners should be engaged in some form of activity which can be observed, although some teachers will argue that learners are already "actively" engaged in the learning process. However, this cannot necessarily be proved unless observable activity is taking place in the learner. Sitting, watching and listening is not enough. In this respect, repetition is also of particular importance in the teaching and learning of skills (including cognitive skills, like problem solving). Learners must be allowed to practice the object skill or skill components within a framework that is meaningful for that skill set. Learners will initially learn to generalise, and then to discriminate the skill so that adaptability of the skill towards any situation is learned. The clinical, behavioural and pharmaceutical skills needed for advancement of extended pharmacy roles can only be learned effectively in this context. The ubiquitous component of most behaviourist approaches involves the notion of reinforcement and, although there are some arguments to the contrary, it is generally held that positive, reward-led reinforcement has a greater impact on learning behaviour than negative, punishment-led reinforcement. It cannot be disputed that reinforcement per se is a prime motivator, whether it be intrinsic reinforcement (self reward) or extrinsic in nature (reward from teachers). Measuring the relative extent of these types of reinforcement has proved to be difficult however, and has detracted from the overall behaviourist argument in learning psychology.

The next principal grouping is the application of cognitive theories of learning psychology to the educational process. Although the groupings are being discussed separately, they all have practical applications which can be utilised in conjunction with other approaches. Learning with understanding is clearly better than learning by rote, or without any measurable level of understanding. As children, we may have learned the alphabet or our arithmetic tables by repetition, with the sole purpose of remembering, for this is the basis of labelling systems which are essential for communication between individuals. There are parts of pharmacy undergraduate curricula which also involve rote learning; the names of types of blood cells or the names of drugs. There is no real reason why a platelet is called a platelet; it is simply a means of common labelling, devoid of any real understanding, which ultimately acts as an aid to understanding via a common terminology. It is important to flag parts of the learning where "labelling" is being presented, as opposed to new concepts which require an understanding.

Within this setting, one key to successful "remembering" (storage and retrieval of useable information) is to present facets of the material as "forceful features". Learners should be aware of these; in other words, they should perceive these features in a context which clearly signals their importance to the learner. If the learners successfully perceive parts of the information as "forceful features" these then become key elements in the knowledge structure of the learner. If presentation and perception of information or concepts are unclear, the learner will have more difficulty in knowledge organisation, even to the point of erroneous structures. Misperception of knowledge or concepts can only be discovered by teacher and learner if interaction takes place between the two, and feedback from learner to teacher is essential if remedial action is required. The sooner this occurs after presenting new material, the more effective this correction will be in avoiding the establishment of erroneous perceptions and erroneous knowledge in the learner. It is necessary that the learner should provide evidence that learning has occurred before cognitive feedback will be of any benefit; post- or in-class questioning, post learning testing, audience response cards, questionnaires, learning diaries are all usable methods for prompting corrective (and reinforcive) feedback. There are obvious overlaps here with the stimulus-response notion of reinforcement, but it is clear that people are more likely to be effective learners if they know how well they are performing.

Most teachers will be able to assign organisation and structure to their teaching; it is debatable whether most of their students would be able to describe this. Evidence suggests that individuals will learn more effectively if they have some idea about the overall structure and framework of a course of learning. The organisation of learning material (the sequencing applied by the teacher) and the structure of the material (the intrinsic logic of the concepts and relationships) are closely related and have obvious importance in any course. Competent teaching may be characterised by organised and structured material, coupled with communication of these aspects to the learners.

The third main grouping of educational principles centres around the personality and social psychological theories, and these have fundamental influences on the teaching method. For instance, we should regard learning as a natural process; as an elemental aspect of human nature, we have a curiosity and a desire to make sense of our surroundings, which provokes a natural propensity for learning. We inherently want to solve problems and make decisions; hence learning is not something exclusive to schools or universities, and all teachers should make efforts to stimulate this innate characteristic of learning. Having said that, we also tend to need a purpose for our actions. To have a purpose is to be able to set goals, or targets, and results in motivation for the learner. Learning cannot be conducted within a vacuum or in an environment that does not recognise or encourage goal setting (personal as well as institutional). A course of learning needs to have aims and objectives which will compliment those of the learner. Curriculum design is an important, and much neglected, attribute in pharmacy undergraduate education which will aid the establishment of common goals for teacher and learner.

Learning is rarely a solitary process and tends to occur most frequently in social situations. Hence group psychology and the internal culture of the learning institution become important modifiers of individual learning effectiveness. The nature of cooperation, the extent of competition, the value systems held by peers and teachers are all fundamental influences on the learning process. Efforts may be needed to change the inherent culture within a particular group of learners, or indeed the teacher group, in order to encourage greater interaction or personal motivation. Coupled with this, significant learning will only occur in non-threatening environments, this being dependent to some extent on the social situation. Positive feedback, reinforcement and the utilisation of natural curiosity are necessary for effective learning and this can realistically only happen in a situation where the learner feels comfortable and stable. To have situations where learners feel threatened to ask (or be asked) questions in lectures or classes, is to have a culture and climate that will not produce motivated and satisfied learners.

Finally, we should spare a thought about responsibility and relevance: relevance is a word increasingly used in pharmacy undergraduate curricula and professional reviews. It is a concept which is becoming more widespread throughout all education, although one suspects that the perception of the meaning within pharmacy is variable. There is no doubt that the future needs of the profession should be the driving force for course content (the "what" of learning) but relevance should also extend to the choice of "how" and "when" for the learner. Significant learning will only take place if the learner chooses how and when to learn. There should be no barrier to designing choice in any course of learning.

In the preceding description, the three main categories of learning theory are presented as separate strands. Several points should be emphasised here; it is clear that these groupings are not mutually exclusive, and most teaching and learning situations will combine aspects of these principles. Teaching utilises a mixture of theories and applications of theories, and no one category can claim to have more or less significance than the others. Successful teaching strategies make use of a wide and full range of applied principles and even the newest teaching methods (see below) utilise these existing theories in an integrated fashion. It is clear that several developments need to be encouraged in higher education if the principles of effective learning are to be fully implemented. Teachers need to ask some searching questions about current teaching practice if progress towards more competent professional graduates is to continue. For instance, how can learners be effective in recognising important features of lectures, presentations or classes if they do not perceive these as being significant? Are the presentations and classes designed in such a way that encoding by the learner is easy (or even possible in some cases)? What is the most efficient use of reinforcers and motivators to encourage more effective learning? Are courses geared up to providing these reinforcers at all? How can teachers help individuals to recognise interpersonal differences in learning and adopt appropriate learning strategies? If these questions are raised more frequently in pharmacy education, then teaching methods may develop to match the educational needs of undergraduates for the role of tomorrow's pharmacists. Many of the traditional teaching methods used in pharmacy education are clearly contradictory to the objectives of some of these learning principles. The lecture for example, may not necessarily engender an active response; it does not facilitate positive feedback, nor does it permit individuality in learning.

PROBLEM-BASED LEARNING

Today's graduates will be practising pharmacy well into the next century. They will have to deal with many fundamental changes in the profession and develop their existing knowledge, acquire new skills and demonstrate competence in a wide range of fields to meet the changing environment. Graduates will thus need to adapt; to self-direct their continuing learning, to develop and participate in change. Problem-based learning may facilitate this. But what is problem-based learning? In many ways it is easier to say what it is not. It is not solving problems or posed questions in class; it is not solving a research problem over the course of a term; it is not class-based project work. Problem-based learning has been a significant development in professional education, and yet is still frequently misunderstood and misquoted. At a fundamental level, problem-based learning is the learning which results from the process of working towards the understanding of a problem.[5] In other words, problem-based learning is about using problems or problematic situations as stimuli to learning, rather than just starting points towards a solution. These problems or problematic situations are considered to be a network or cluster of interrelated problems and contextual conditions. It is a concept of knowledge, understanding and education very different from the more usual subject orientated approach (Table 2).

TABLE 2

Problem based learning process can be identified by:

- Cumulative learning: Repeated reintroduction of subjects across a broad range, with increasing sophistication whenever it may contribute to the problematic situation.

- Integrated learning: All subjects available for study as required by a problem.

- Progression: As the learners mature, the curriculum should change and progress.

- Consistency: The learning must be supported throughout the curriculum and curriculum implementation.

With a subject orientation to education, as traditional in pharmacy, expertise is regarded as "knowing a lot", to possess knowledge about content, to have "covered" a lot during one's education. A general tendency is for propositional knowledge, a knowledge that "x is this" or "y is that". In fairness, it is true to say that in professional practice one needs knowledge of how to do something, but much vocational education is also primarily concerned with content and propositional knowledge as the main means of equipping future professionals.

Expertise can also be equated with an understanding of problems and problematic situations together with an ability to identify components of these problems and knowledge of how to solve them. Problem-based learning does not ignore the importance of content, but it does ignore the belief that content is best acquired in an abstract manner, in large quantities, in propositional form, and should only be later "applied in real life" once it has been thoroughly "learned" at university. Problem-based learning is an integrated process, meaning an integration of "knowing what" with "knowing how". This process commences with establishing what needs to be known in order to manage a problem; hence starting with the problem "X" (or problematic situation "X") and learning "backwards" from that point, rather than the traditional process of first acquiring knowledge about A, B, C and D as a prerequisite to addressing problem X. A carefully designed problem-based learning course will have the following effects on learners:

i.   Encouragement of open minded approaches to learning, involving self-direction and critical appraisal. This may be summarised perhaps as "active learning".
ii. The process acknowledges the learner and the teacher as different individuals, whilst creating a framework that has common purpose for both. This modifies the usual teacher–student relationship in higher education.
iii. The process reflects the nature of knowledge as complex, interrelated and changeable. It recognises the needs of communities (societies, cultures) as well as those of individuals.

For these, and other reasons, problem-based learning is perceived by many as a threatening philosophy. It may also generate considerable anxiety in terms of appraisal of students, appraisal of courses, disruption of work patterns and engender resistance to change. However, problem-based learning produces competent individuals: graduates who are adaptable and motivated to continually learn and who will promote and facilitate change.

TEACHING PHARMACY PRACTICE IN A PROBLEM-BASED DESIGN

At the School of Pharmacy, University of London, we have been experimenting with two forms of educational strategy; systems education methodology as applied to the third year of pharmacy practice study, and a competency based system of learning for the first two years of study. We shall argue the case for this latter method of learning, and the outcomes that may result.

Learning Philosophy

The Pharmacy Practice course for the first and second year of study is divided into three levels. These represent a graded organisation of material and learning skills which increase in complexity as learners progress through them. The course has been conceived as a means to enable and ensure personal progression by design rather than serendipity. Learners are thus expected to demonstrate personal competence at each level before progressing onwards. The learning that students complete, and the work that they produce during these three levels, form the basis of the Third Year of study. At this stage, skills-orientated learning (learning based on acquiring thinking and behavioural or manipulative experience/practice) enable students to approach more specialised topics.

We believe it is important that learners perceive the Pharmacy Practice course as a continuing education throughout the three years; it is not designed or intended to be compartmentalised. Learners will identify the need to employ knowledge and skills from other areas of study during the course, even though at the present time, these other areas remain essentially subject-led.

Classes are organised around Working Groups of six learners, with each individual responsible to the other Group members for progress through the modules of an exercise. To facilitate this learning culture, a purpose built laboratory encourages the performance of the Working Groups as self-contained, fully resourced units. The unit size of six is identified as an optimal small group size in terms of learning efficiency and the latter is enhanced by seating the Group members at "hexagonal" work benches designed with the learning principles outlined earlier in mind; a relevant environment being essential for learner satisfaction. As a direct consequence of this course design, learners rapidly perceive the need for, and develop the means to, ensure good communications within the Group. Thus learning becomes a shared experience, with tutors encouraging each individual to reach their full potential.

The learning experiences are problem-based. In general, this requires learners to discover for themselves what they need to learn, rather than be instructed by tutors, whose role is to provide guidance and to facilitate personal development. Problem-based learning in this context relies on the setting and achievement of objectives, with the specificity of the objectives defining the level or competence of the knowledge or skill concerned. Learners are appraised on how and when they achieve the stated objectives, a process which then becomes a personal competence indicator.

Appraisal

The Exercises and the learning experiences they contain mandate appraisal to satisfy educational principles. In essence, appraisal acts as a monitor of personal progress, as a measure of the effectiveness of a particular individual's learning and as an indicator of learning or behavioural difficulties that the individual may experience. In the system outlined here, individuals who encounter problems are rapidly identified by the teaching team. Early intervention then enables the achievement of full learning potential. The net result is that learners know how much and how well they are learning – a basic process in education.

Appraisal of the learners is based on a criterion referenced method. This type of appraisal is concerned with how an individual has performed, independent of the achievements of others. The usual practice of giving a mark (8/10, 14/20, etc) is only meaningful when an individual's performance is considered in the context of the whole class. This is the process of norm-referenced marking. Criterion referenced evaluation is based on clear cut-off points, and is therefore related to a level of competence. The advantages of this system are clear; individuals know what constitutes an acceptable learning outcome and can identify when further learning is necessary. The implementation of this type of appraisal is linked with the use of learning objectives and learning profiles, and each module therefore starts with a set of objectives which are appraised before any new experience commences. Throughout the course, each set of competencies is marked by student self-assessment and tutor assessment.

Outcome Measures

Preliminary evaluation of the course indicates that students adapt to this method of learning very quickly. It may be acceptable because it is introduced within two weeks of commencing their degree. Appraisals have been collated for 103 students over a two year period ending July 1993. This sample population represents the first cohort of learners to progress through the new course design. The total number of variables measured for each student was approximately 1500, with each variable representing a dichotomous assessment of competency. The general measure used is the "percent correct" mark. This is derived by expressing the sum of the variables in which "competency" is achieved as a percentage of the maximum number of "competencies" that could be attained by the student. A percent (%) mark can then be calculated for each individual variable or group of variables as a function of time. The result is that a dichotomous measure of competency in specified categories is converted into a percentage number of "correct" competencies, termed the "percent correct" mark. This is a common procedure for calculating scores from a criterion referenced system of marking.

In general, students tend to mark themselves higher than tutors. This may be contradictory to norm-referenced systems, where evidence suggests that student and tutor marks often turn out to be very similar.[6,7] Student marks overall remain higher than tutor marks ($p < 0.001$), although this difference is not seen at the start of the course. The discrepancy between tutor and student assessment is expected because of the nature of the marking scheme: competencies are being assessed, and the purpose of the teaching and learning is to highlight non-competent skills. Tutors would be expected to recognise non-competency before students. This is interpreted as the students gaining in confidence with their performance, whilst tutors are still expected to detect deficiencies. Students tend to assess their performance as improving through the course and, at the same time, it is noted that the tutor % correct marks also increase (start of course compared to end p<0.001), meaning that students do indeed improve their competencies overall. This result suggests that the basic premise of the learning (and marking) system is justified. Students get better according to their tutors, and also are able to assess this improvement themselves. However, the "gap" between tutor and student scores suggests that for this type of learning methodology, self-assessment on its own is not the most appropriate measure of ability, and that tutor-based monitoring is essential for learning success. However, it is noted that the gap between student and tutor assessments tends to diminish towards the end of the course towards a non-significant difference, although the general trend is for all scores to increase. Increasingly, it seems, student and tutor scores converge as students improve their learning and self-assessment skills.

In summary, students performed self-assessment by comparing their own performance against a standard set of competencies, within a framework of learning objectives. Overall, students improve as measured by a % correct score for these competencies, and this is reflected in both tutor and self-assessed scores. Students tend to assess their personal competencies higher compared to tutors, and this is interpreted as a gain in self-confidence, but also as evidence that problem-based learning, using competency assessment, needs skilled tutors to monitor students progress effectively and safely.

We are confident that learners are developing problem solving skills and are assertive in their approach to learning and data acquisition, more so than that engendered by traditional method of teaching pharmacy practice.

CONCLUSION

For teachers of pharmacy, an understanding of learning theories, and the adaptation and inclusion of these theories in the design of learning, is a basic requirement for undergraduate education. An understanding of the learning process however, is probably not enough, and the need for curriculum design cannot be overstated. The haphazard and arbitrary inclusion of new ideas of learning theory into a course is unlikely to improve undergraduate and subsequent post-graduate behaviour.

We describe a problem-based learning method which is being used in conjunction with assessments of competency, where emphasis is not on acquisition of knowledge, but on deciding what knowledge and skills are needed to solve problems and then practising and developing these. The problems or problematic stimuli reflect the nature of problems encountered in the work place. The setting of learning objectives, increasing in complexity throughout the course, and building on previous learning allows the learner to have a clear idea of where she or he is heading. Competency based assessments allow learners to monitor their own progress, without being compared to one another. Pharmacists must be equipped with the skills, motivation and desire to adapt to changing health care needs. It is at undergraduate level that educational processes can change behaviour to produce professionals with the skills and motivation for problem solving and life-long learning.

REFERENCES

1. Skinner BF. *The behaviour of organisms.* New York: Appleton-Century-Crofts; 1938.
2. Blackman D. Images of man in contemporary behaviourism. In: Chapman AJ, Jones DM. eds. *Models of man.* Leicester: British Psychological Society; 1980.
3. Herzberg F. *Work and nature of man.* Cleveland, Ohio: World Publishing; 1966.
4. Hilgard ER, Bower G. *Theories of Learning,* 4th ed. Englewood Cliffs, New Jersey: Prentice Hall; 1975.
5. Barrows HS, Tamblyn RM. *Problem-Based Learning: An Approach to Medical education.* New York: Springer; 1980.
6. Boud DJ. *Self and peer assessment in higher and continuing professional education: An annotated bibliography.* Occasional Publication No. 16. Sydney: tertiary Education Research Centre, University of South Wales; 1980.
7. Orpen C. Student v lecturer assessment of learning: a research note. *Higher Education* 1992; 11: 567-72.

CHAPTER SIXTEEN

FROM VOCATIONAL TRAINING TO ACADEMIC DISCIPLINE: A BRIEF COMMENT ON SOCIAL PHARMACY IN SWEDEN

Kerstin Bingefors and Dag Isacson

INTRODUCTION

The professional role of the pharmacist has changed markedly during the past three decades. The large scale development of the pharmaceutical industry, increasing production of prepackaged medicines and the subsequent decline in compounding as a major task within pharmacy has created a sense of bewilderment among pharmacists (see also chapter 2). Indeed, the profession's response to change has been addressed by several commentators.[1-6]

Social pharmacy is generally defined as the interface between pharmacy and society and is important in preparing graduates for practice in a rapidly changing world.[7] Unfortunately, from its inception in Sweden in the early seventies, social pharmacy has served to preserve an obsolete professional role rather than facilitate the individual and professional development of pharmacy graduates. Social pharmacy in Sweden then, was a relic of the earlier vocational school training of pharmacists. It occupied a large part of the undergraduate curriculum, where students devoted an inordinate amount of time to learning basic pharmacy procedures, many of which were outdated within 6 to 12 months after graduation. Under the auspices of "Social Pharmacy" considerable time was given over to political indoctrination. The "proper" opinions varied with lecturers' political opinions. In the middle of the seventies the teaching was right wing, while at the beginning of the eighties the teaching was very left wing. With no scientific base, social pharmacy was considered by the students as a rather meaningless subject in the undergraduate program. A revision of the curriculum in the early eighties however, resulted in a new philosophy underpinning social pharmacy in Sweden.

CURRICULUM DEVELOPMENT AND NEEDS ASSESSMENT

In curriculum development it is essential to define the desired outcomes, i.e. which abilities should the graduate possess after completing their course. These abilities, in turn, should be defined on the basis of a need for particular competencies in professional practice. In our case, we not only had to design an undergraduate curriculum but also create a scientific foundation for social pharmacy.

When assessing the educational needs of pharmacists, two different perspectives were considered – that of the patient, and that of the population at large. In respect of the patients' perspective we focused on the salient characteristics of those who present to the pharmacy: their drug usage, morbidity patterns and prognoses. We then considered what knowledge and skills are needed to give optimal pharmaceutical services to these patients.

An epidemiological approach was used to yield a population perspective of pharmaceutical services. We also concentrated on pharmacists' collaboration with other health professionals and the impact of pharmacists on public health. As an example, Figure 1 shows the proportion of the population in a Swedish community who used at least one prescription drug in 1986. This is the basis of

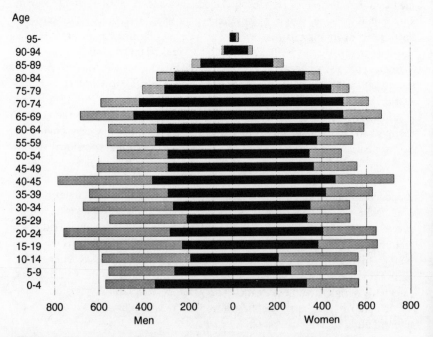

Figure 1: The proportion of the population in a Swedish community using at least one prescription drug (black) during 1986, by sex and age.

pharmacy intervention in the community. If we add clients who buy over-the-counter medicines, it is evident that the pharmacy has contacts with a majority of the population each year.

We can conclude that the pharmacist is a potentially very important source both for implementing a more rational use of drugs and for public health interventions in the community. Consequently, the educational focus should be on the need for adequate training in order to fulfil these aims. Notwithstanding this, many Schools of Pharmacy continue to place considerable emphasis on natural sciences, while minimising the social and behavioural parts of the curriculum.

Using the previously mentioned needs assessment, combined with a review of other curricula for health professionals we decided on Public Health, Health Services Research, Pharmacoepidemiology and Health Economics as the conceptual and methodological foundation for Social Pharmacy (Figure 2). In combination with the pharmaceutical sciences and communication skills, this would provide the graduate with a groundwork for developing what is now known as "Pharmaceutical Care" in his/her future practice.

TEACHING METHODS

Pharmaceutical education has traditionally relied on classical teaching methods, especially that of rote learning. Critics of these approaches maintain that they do not facilitate personal development. The problem based curriculum (based upon Kolb's experiential learning theory[8]) was subsequently developed in response to such criticisms.[9,10] However, a completely problem based

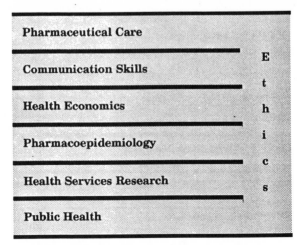

Figure 2: Social Pharmacy as a multidisciplinary area within pharmacy education.

curriculum is heavily resource dependent and we have adapted the methods to meet our particular needs and available resources. (For a fuller exposition of the application of teaching methods to social pharmacy see chapter 15).

Social pharmacy is now project based with students working in groups, on topics in public health with an emphasis on the role of pharmacy. They are offered lectures, seminars and laboratory sessions in methodology and are free to collect information from a range of sources, including computerised data bases, libraries and other university departments. The resulting report has to be of sufficient quality for them to use as teaching material for their own teaching sessions.

RESEARCH

Social Pharmacy, as defined in Sweden, covers a very broad field and it is important to develop competencies in selected areas commensurate with available expertise. The major areas of research within the division of Social Pharmacy in Sweden, have focused on Pharmaceutical and Health Services research and Pharmacoepidemiology, and in particular on the use of psychotropic drugs, drug use among the elderly, use of small scale preparations and heavy users of prescription drugs. Research students on the PhD program within the division are also encouraged to attend research courses in related fields such as medical statistics, public health, epidemiology, medical sociology, ethics and health economics.

THE FUTURE OF SOCIAL PHARMACY

The profession of pharmacy and pharmaceutical education will most certainly undergo further changes in the near future.[11-13] A Social Pharmacy curriculum which equips graduates for lifelong learning and development will be increasingly important. Such a steadily evolving discipline requires high quality education and a research base which is of interest to professionals outside of pharmacy. For a relatively new component of pharmaceutical education, social pharmacy in Sweden has come a long way in a relatively short time, though its continual development is crucial to equip undergraduates for practice in future decades.

REFERENCES

1. Birenbaum A. Reprofessionalisation in Pharmacy. *Social Science and Medicine* 1982; 16: 871-878.
2. Denzin NK, Mettlin CJ. Incomplete professionalisation: the case of pharmacy. *Social Forces* 1968; 46: 375-381.

3. Herman McCormack T. The druggists' dilemma: Problems of a marginal occupation. *American Journal of Sociology* 1956; 61: 308-315.
4. Holloway SWF, Jewson ND, Mason DJ. "Reprofessionalisation" or "occupational imperialism?": Some reflections on pharmacy in Britain. *Social Science and Medicine* 1986; 23: 323-332.
5. Labreche DG. The rise and fall of the apothecary: Will history repeat itself? *Pharmacotherapy* 1989; 2: 105-111.
6. Sanazaro PJ. Medicine and pharmacy: Our once and future status as professionals. *American Journal of Hospital Pharmacy* 1987; 44: 521-524.
7. Harding G, Taylor KMG. Defining Social Pharmacy. *International Journal of Pharmacy Practice* 1993; 2: 62-63.
8. Kolb D. *Experiential learning* 1st ed. Englewood Cliffs: Prentice-Hall Inc.; 1984.
9. Barrows H. A taxonomy of problem-based learning methods. *Medical Education* 1986; 20: 481-486.
10. Neufeld V, Barrows H. "The McMaster philosophy": An approach to medical education. *Journal of Medical Education* 1974; 49: 1040-1050.
11. Trinca CE. Pharmacy in the 21st Century: Introductory comments. *American Journal of Pharmaceutical Education* 1989; 53(suppl): 6s-7s.
12. Strand L, Cipolle R, Morley P, Perrier D. Levels of pharmaceutical care: A needs-based approach. *American Journal of Hospital Pharmacy* 1991; 48: 547-550.
13. Ebert R. Health professions education for year 2001. *American Journal of Pharmaceutical Education* 1991; 55: 356-360.

INDEX